Collaborator:

Donna L. Frownfelter, A.B., R.P.T., A.R.I.T.
Director of Respiratory Rehabilitation
Rush-Presbyterian-St. Luke's Hospital
Chicago, Illinois

Photographers:

Vicki Catalani

The late Edwin Bonk

Beard's

MASSAGE

Principles and Techniques

Elizabeth C. Wood, A.M., M.S., R.P.T.

Formerly, Associate Professor of Physical Therapy
Department of Rehabilitation Medicine
Northwestern University Medical School
Chicago, Illinois

SECOND EDITION

W. B. SAUNDERS COMPANY, Philadelphia, London, Toronto

W. B. Saunders Company: West Washington Square
Philadelphia, Pa. 19105

12 Dyott Street
London, WC1A 1DB

833 Oxford Street
Toronto, Ontario M8Z 5T9, Canada

Beard's Massage

ISBN   0-7216-9591-4

Last digit is the print number: 9   8   7   6   5   4   3   2

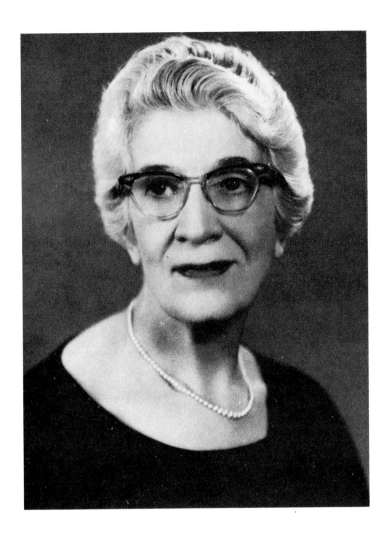

This book is dedicated to the memory
of

GERTRUDE BEARD, R.N, R.P.T.

My colleague and friend, without
whom there would have been no First
Edition.

preface

Much of the Second Edition of this textbook remains essentially unchanged from the First Edition. The history, basic principles and techniques of massage do not change greatly in ten years.

However, because of the increased use in the United States of massage procedures for the care of patients with respiratory problems, some major changes and additions have been made in Chapter 3, Principles of Massage, Chapter 4, Effects of Massage, and Chapter 5, Techniques. New material has been added to Chapter 1, and Chapter 4, after a review of the recent literature.

The title of this edition—*Beard's Massage: Principles and Techniques*—emphasizes Gertrude Beard's (1887–1971) major contributions to the book. The dedication to her, and the retention from the First Edition of the Foreword by Dr. Paul B. Magnuson (1884–1968) honor these two pioneers in the fields of physical therapy and rehabilitation for their dedication to physical therapy students and to patients over a period of fifty years.

The techniques for general massage follow rather closely a Swedish massage system learned by Miss Beard from Minna Schmidt of Philadelphia, before the Hoffa methods were widely used in the United States. The local massage techniques follow quite closely the modified Hoffa method taught at Children's Hospital in Boston by Janet B. Merrill, under the direction of Dr. Robert W. Lovett and his successor, Dr. Arthur T. Legg.

The material on principles and techniques of massage for patients with respiratory problems is the work of my colleague Mrs. Donna L. Frownfelter, a specialist in chest physical therapy. She has spent three years in respiratory therapy and four years in chest physical therapy at Northwestern Memorial Hospital (Wesley Pavilion) in Chicago, the last two years as Chief Chest Physical Therapist. In July, 1973, she became Director of Respiratory Rehabilitation at Rush-Presbyterian—St. Luke's Hospital in Chicago. She is also Instructor in Physical Therapy at both Northwestern University Medical School and Chicago Medical School/University of Health Sciences. It has been a pleasure, a privilege and a stimulating experience to work with her in the preparation of this new edition.

I gratefully acknowledge the services of Vicki Catalani and the late Edwin Bonk, photographers, in taking the photographs used in this book. I thank Robert F. Benway, Instructor, Northwestern University Affiliated School of Respiratory Therapy at Northwestern Memorial Hospital, for acting as patient in the illustrations on percussion and vibration techniques and postural drainage; also Karen Streubing, R.N., B.S.N., and the Northern Illinois Chapter of the National Cystic Fibrosis Research Foundation for allowing us to include their instructions and drawings (by Todd R. Riddell, D.D.S.) on postural drainage, including those for small babies.

My thanks go once again to some 700 graduates of Northwestern University's Course in Physical Therapy, who helped in evaluating both content and various methods of presenting this material while they were students.

Brian C. Decker of the W. B. Saunders Company has been most helpful in advising on the preparation of this new edition and in seeing to the execution of the exacting details of production required for such a book as this. One could not ask for any greater cooperation and assistance than he and his staff have given.

ELIZABETH C. WOOD

foreword
to the first edition

There are some things in every man's life that have a great effect upon his future success and the success of some of the people around him. One of these things happened to me when a physical therapist named Gertrude Beard came to Chicago shortly after the First World War, after she was discharged from the Army.

Miss Beard was taken onto the staff of Wesley Hospital immediately and started work on my patients, most of them workers who had been injured at the stockyards. She worked in a place called the "bath department," which consisted of one shower, one Scotch douche, a table and a couple of sinks. She and the patients had to sit on stools, and no one in the hospital took her appearance with any great degree of hope that she was going to do anything that had not been done before. At that time (1919–1920) physical therapy, in my experience, was something to do when you couldn't think of anything else to do to get rid of the patient.

Miss Beard had made a study of what was not considered a very great science at that time, and went on to develop physical therapy techniques which have brought help to many patients who would never have recovered had it not been for her efforts.

In 1927 she became the technical director of Northwestern University's new school of physical therapy. She and her teaching colleagues have taught more than five hundred physical therapists the techniques and principles of physical therapy since that date. The story of their work is worth noting – a story of devoted, dedicated persons who believe in what they know, and who continue to educate doctors and patients as well as students in the benefits of physical therapy and especially massage.

Massage has often been neglected in favor of other physical measures which can be used more easily. Massage requires skilled use of the hands and brain for its curative effects – producing or regaining elasticity of tissues, stimulating blood supply, giving the patient confidence and at the same time giving him encouragement and psychological stimulation to use the part that is disabled – and no machine can substitute. There is a psychology that goes along with any form of medical treatment, and if the physical therapist is not using his or her powers of encouragement to get the patient to do what he should do, then he or she is not doing a job in whatever is being done.

In my opinion massage is one of the things that can be neglected, misused, paid for and thrown out the window without accomplishing what it should unless it is understood and properly applied. This book presents a clear picture of techniques and the principles upon which they are based. The text is well written and illustrated and should be read and reread by the doctor and the physical therapist to the everlasting benefit of the patient's recovery.

PAUL B. MAGNUSON, M.D.
Professor of Bone and Joint Surgery,
Emeritus, Northwestern University
Medical School
Founder and Honorary Chairman,
Rehabilitation Institute of Chicago
Former Chief Medical Director, Veterans
Administration

May 1964

contents

APPENDIX 1

APPENDIX 2

BIBLIOGRAPHY

INDEX

chapter 1

introduction

The word massage means "to knead" and is the term used to designate certain manipulations of the soft tissues of the body; these manipulations are most effectively performed with the hands and are administered for the purpose of producing effects on the nervous, muscular, and respiratory systems and the local and general circulation of the blood and lymph.

Many mechanical devices have been developed as substitutes for human hands in the application of massage. However, the sensation of touch which exists in the hands conveys information that is essential for the intelligent application of massage. The reaction of the tissues to the treatment should be observed with an understanding of the anatomy, physiology, and pathology of the tissues under treatment, so as to vary each maneuver according to the needs of the moment. No mechanical device can obtain such information or satisfactorily substitute for well-trained human hands directed by the judgment of an intelligent therapist.

Massage is one of the oldest forms of treatment for human ills. Over the centuries it has been referred to in history, literature, and art, as well as in medicine. Many claims have been made for its efficacy for many and varied conditions, and persons with many and varied qualifications have prescribed and performed massage.

Various systems and techniques have been developed, as well as some rationale (other than a "laying on of hands") for the use of massage in treating patients.

James B. Mennell (1880–1957), physician at St. Thomas's Hospital in London, has had a great influence on the use of massage in present-day practice in England and the United States. His rational and conservative principles were based on his study with Just Lucas-Championnière and his own practice in the treatment of fractures. From these experiences he recognized the value of careful, gentle massage, in contrast to some of the vigorous and painful massage advocated by other physicians in the early part of the twentieth century (see Table VII, p. 32–35). These principles, expressed in his writings and in his personal comments to Gertrude Beard, are often referred to in this book, especially in Chapters 3 and 4.

To be recognized as professionally competent in the application of massage the nurse, physical therapist, physical therapist assistant, or respiratory (inhalation) therapist must be trained in an accredited educational program recognized by the medical and other professions as adequate to meet professional standards.

The therapist who gives massage must know human anatomy and physiology. He must understand the relationship between the structure and function of the tissues being treated and the total function of the patient. He must know pathology, so that he can understand how to use massage to obtain the effects that are desired to alleviate the pathological condition being treated. He must be skilled in the proper manipulations of tissues, so that he can accomplish this aim and at the same time not cause further damage to the tissues or harm to the patient.

As a professional person, he should be indoctrinated in professional ethics, so that he is aware of his responsibilities to both physician and patient in promoting the patient's welfare. To this end, he should foster good patient-physician as well as patient-therapist rapport and work closely with the physician who prescribes the treatment.

The therapist should maintain a professional attitude in all his relations with patients. He should possess poise and dignity. His speech and manner should always be courteous. Conversation should be guarded, and avoided when the patient wishes to rest.

Immaculate personal cleanliness on the part of any person working with patients is essential because of the close contact which he has with the patient. Body odors are indications of ill health or careless personal hygiene and are particularly offensive.

The uniform should be neat and clean and allow for free movement of the arms and shoulders. The shoes should be comfortable, with low or moderate heels. The hair should be neatly groomed. No jewelry should be worn, with the exception of a watch, a professional pin, and perhaps a plain wedding ring.

The therapist's hands should be soft, warm, and dry with nails clean, not too long, and free from rough hangnails. Colored nail polish should not be used. The hands should be washed in the presence of the patient, or with his knowledge, before beginning treatment and, if the face is to be included, washed again before massaging the face.

In addition to adequate professional training, a therapist should have a personality which enables him to deal with sick or handicapped individuals. Unselfishness, patience, a spirit of loyalty to the patient, an interest in his welfare, and the ability to express this in a thoughtful and practical manner are essential.

Massage is used in many cases that require treatment over a protracted period. The time required for return of function may be long and tedious, and a patient is often beset with periods of discouragement. Evidence of interest in the patient's welfare, an attitude of kindness, a cheerful manner, an ability to point out encouraging signs of progress make it possible for the therapist to gain the confidence and cooperation of the patient and to motivate him to continue to strive for recovery.

The purpose of this book is to give some historical perspective for understanding the use of massage and its development; to present basic principles related to administering massage treatment; to consider what is known, and unknown, concerning the effects of massage; and to describe basic techniques for general and local massage procedures.

Discussion of the use of massage procedures for the treatment of specific diagnoses (e.g., arthritis, "low back" syndrome, strokes, fractures) is deliberately omitted. The therapist's knowledge of anatomy, physiology and pathology, and his knowledge of the effects which can be expected from the various types of massage properly applied will enable him to discuss with the prescribing physician what massage may or may not be suitable for each patient being treated. (See Chap. III, p. 36–37.)

Since World War II there has been a decrease in the amount of massage treatment being prescribed by many physicians, perhaps because giving massage is always time consuming and requires not only real skill but sometimes strenuous output of effort on the part of the therapist. The basis for prescribing massage is still largely empiric rather than scientific. Nevertheless, many physical therapists, physicians and patients are convinced by clinical experience that massage has therapeutic value if basic principles are followed and the massage is skillfully done.

A 1966–67 survey of 260 physical therapists and facilities on current trends in the use of therapeutic massage[64] showed that of the 169 replies to a questionnaire 92 per cent believed in its value, while 8 per cent said they did not. Reasons given for its frequent use were relaxation, psychological effects, effects on circulation, reduction of edema, analgesic effect, stretching of adhesions and value of personal contact. Other reasons offered included gaining of knowledge of the physical state of tissues (via palpation for muscle tone, fibrotic nodules and lipomas), facilitating muscular effort by the patient and encouraging the patient to return for further treatment. Reasons for not using massage were listed as too time consuming, not sufficient time for therapist to treat adequately, other methods of treatment (such as electrical stimulation, heat, and ultra sound) more effective, no benefits other than temporary comfort observed. Veterans Administration and military hospitals seldom use massage, according to this survey.

chapter 2

a history of massage technique

Massage is mentioned as a form of treatment in the earliest medical records, and its use continues down through history. Writings of physicians, philosophers, poets, and historians show that some form of rubbing or anointing was used among both savage and civilized nations from the most ancient times.

Hippocrates (460–380 B.C.),[19, 35] in discussing the treatment of a dislocated shoulder following reduction, said, "And it is necessary to rub the shoulder gently and smoothly. The physician must be experienced in many things, but assuredly also in rubbing; for things that have the same name have not the same effects. For rubbing can bind a joint which is too loose and loosen a joint that is too hard. However, a shoulder in the condition described should be rubbed with soft hands and, above all things, gently; but the joint should be moved about, not violently, but so far as it can be done without producing pain."

In much written medical history, massage and exercises are referred to simultaneously, and in the very early literature there is little distinction between the two. Kleen (1847–1923) of Sweden, who published a handbook of massage in 1895, claims to be the first to show clearly that massage is not an exercise therapy.

In reviewing the literature on massage, one is impressed with the lack of detailed description. Even in some rather recent research, there is little information on the actual technique. When one observes the great variance in the massage techniques used today and the frequent apparent lack of scientific basis for the movements that are given, one wonders how any conclusions can be made as to their value or lack of value in treatment. The lack of detailed information on techniques and the confusion in the meaning of the current modern terms has led to this study of the literature. It is not a complete account of the history of massage. Only the techniques are considered and a comparison of the methods made to determine, if possible, their influence upon the development of present-day methods and techniques. Much of the information on the early history of massage as presented in this study has been obtained from the publications of Graham (1848–1928), Bucholz (1874–(?)1942), Coulter (1885–1949), and others. The study has been comprehensive, but a complete survey of the literature has not been attempted.

DEFINITIONS OF MASSAGE

The early medical literature is devoid of any comprehensive definition of massage. A medical dictionary of 1880[72] offers this: "Massage, from the Greek, meaning to knead. Signifying the act of shampooing."

William Murrell (1853–1912) of Edinburgh and London, writing at about the same time, was at once less general and more specific when he defined massage as "the scientific mode of treating certain forms of a disease by systematic manipulations." He, you will note, limited massage to the amelioration of disease but evidently realized the need for a system in its use. He placed no limit on means of massage. At the same time, Douglas Graham, of Boston, writing from 1884 to 1918, called massage "a term now generally accepted by European and American physicians to signify a group of procedures which are usually done with the hands, such as friction, kneading, manipulations, rolling, and percussion of the external tissues of the body in a variety of ways, either with a curative, palliative, or hygienic object in view." He went much further than Murrell (in recognizing that there was a term needing a definition) and limited the means to the hand, the surfaces involved to the external tissues, and the objective as being curative, palliative, or hygienic.

E. A. G. Kleen of Sweden,[42] contemporary with Graham's early works, limited the areas involved to the soft tissues. To the hand, as a means, he added apparatus. This seems inconsistent, since he eliminated the idea that massage is exercise. In this he differed from his early compatriot, Peter H. Ling (1776–1839), also of Sweden.[41]

Albert Hoffa (1859–1907) of Germany also limited the means of massage to the hand but was more embracing in its field of use. He applied it to all the "mechanical procedures that can cure illness."[8]

At about the same time, another German J. B. Zabludowski (1851–1906), also limited the means to the hand but specified "skillful hand grasps, skillfully and systematically applied to the body." While limiting the movement to skillful hand grasps he, like Murrell, recognized the use of systems.

C. Herman Bucholz, of the United States (Boston) and Germany, was as indefinite as any of his early predecessors. He did not mention the hand or any other means in his recommended manipulation of the soft tissues for therapeutic purposes.

Even James B. Mennell (1880–1957), whose great contributions have made the science of massage what it is today—even he gave no formal definition.

In 1932, John S. Coulter (1885–1949) said, "According to the present generally accepted meaning of the word, massage includes a great number of manipulations of the tissues and organs of the body for therapeutic purposes."

In 1952, Gertrude Beard defined massage as stated in the opening sentence of Chapter 1. The definition is repeated here:

Massage is the term used to designate certain manipulations of the soft tissues of the body; these manipulations are most effectively performed with the hands, and are administered for the purpose of producing effects on the nervous, muscular and respiratory systems and the local and general circulation of the blood and lymph.

The author regards this definition as comprehensive, expressing the manner and purpose of this form of treatment.

TERMINOLOGY OF MASSAGE
(See table I on pages 15–21)

A student of the literature must be impressed with the number of different terms used for the movements of massage over the years. Although similarities exist, there is considerable confusion, and a comparison will reveal that few writers have given the same meanings to these terms. A survey of these differences seems necessary if one is to be able to interpret correctly any reading of earlier massage techniques and at the same time possess a clear idea of the meanings presently accepted.

There is a similarity in the terms used by the various advocates of massage among the ancient Greeks and Romans from the time of Homer (ninth century B.C.) through the fourth and fifth centuries A.D. "Friction," "rubbing," and "anointing" were used most frequently by these writers. Celsus, of Rome (25 B.C.–50 A.D.),[30] used, in addition, the term "unction." "Anatripis" and "rubbing" were the terms used by Hippocrates of Greece;[35] later Galen (131–200 A.D.) of Rome adopted the term "anatripsis" from Hippocrates but added the terms "tripsis," "tripsisparaskeulasthke," and "apotherapeia." Oribasius (325–403 A.D.),[30] a Roman who followed Galen a century later, described apotherapeia as "bathing," "friction," and "inunction." Other terms used in this period were "pommeling," "squeezing," and "pinching."

There is little literature on medical practice during the Dark Ages, but we find the terminology of the earlier period is carried over by the users of massage during the fifteenth, sixteenth, and seventeenth centuries in many of the European countries.

Among these writers were the noted surgeon, Ambroise Paré (1518–1590),[30] of France, and the famous physician Thomas Sydenham (1624–1689),[30] of England. They confined the terminology to "friction." P. Alpinus (1553–1617),[30] of Italy, used "rubbing" but added "maxalation," "manipulation," and "pressure"; Frederick Hoffman (1660–1742),[30, 35] of Prussia, adopted Galen's term "apotherapeia." Hieronymus Fabricius (1537–1619),[30] an Italian, seems to be the first to have used the term "kneading," and he also used "rubbing."

In the early part of the nineteenth century there was a definite change in terminology, evidently due to the influence of Peter Ling[30, 37] of Sweden. Ling, to whom credit has been given as the originator of the Swedish system of massage, traveled widely over all Europe and incorporated the use of the French terms "effleurage," "pétrissage," "massage á friction," and "tapotement" into his system. To these he added "rolling," "slapping," "pinching," "shaking," "vibration," and "joint movement," a specific example of including a part of present-day exercise in the classification of massage movements. Johann Mezger (1839–1909),[6] of Holland, used the French terminology exclusively, and William Beveridge (1774–1839),[35] of Scotland, seems to be original in his use of the term "finger rubbing." Lucas-Championnière (1843–1913),[54] of France, was also unique in his terminology; his gentle massage, which he termed "glucokinesis" and "effrayante," has greatly influenced the massage technique of present times.

The terms used by the islanders of Tonga in this same period were "Toogi-Toogi," "Mili," and "Fota"; while the Hawaiians used "lomi-lomi."[30]

In the early twentieth century, medical men in the United States contributed to the literature of massage. Graham avoided the French terms and listed "friction, kneading, manipulation, rolling, pinching, percussion, movement, pressure, squeezing" and the very early Italian term "maxalation." J. H. Kellogg (1852–1943), of Battle Creek, Michigan, described 37 different movements, as contrasted to some of the English writers of a century earlier, for example, John Grosvenor (1742–1823),[18, 30] who used only "friction."

Murrell of Scotland and England, Kleen of Sweden, Hoffa of Germany, Bucholz of Germany and the United States, and John K. Mitchell (1859–1917) of the United States held to the French terminology, while Zabludowski of Germany and Mennell of England dropped it almost entirely.

Kleen, Zabludowski, Mitchell, Bucholz, and Mennell gave a rather simple general classification of the terminology with subdivisions of the movements. Mennell's general classification was stroking, compression, and percussion.

There is much confusion in the contemporary terminology. Louisa L. Despard (in 1932) and Frances Tappan (in 1961) continue to use a mixture of French and English terms.

It is difficult to trace any precise development of the terminology of massage as it is used today. Certainly Ling had an influence by his introduction of the French terms,[37, 56] and although there is a trend by modern authors to discontinue their use, they do exist even in current literature.

DESCRIPTION OF MASSAGE MOVEMENTS

There is little description of the massage movements in the early literature. The author has limited analysis of the description of the movements to the available information since the time of Ling and the terms to those most commonly used today, namely: pétrissage, kneading, friction, effleurage, and stroking. Tapotement, vibration, and shaking have changed very little in meaning; therefore, they will not be included.

In order to interpret the meaning of the terms used by various authors, it is necessary to analyze the following aspects of the technique: direction of the movement, amount of pressure applied, the part of the hand used in performing the movement, the actual motion that is performed, and the specific tissues of the body to which it is applied.

Petrissage
(See Table II on pages 22 and 23)

To perform pétrissage, Ling[37] grasped the tissues between the thumb and fingers while Mitchell, Kellogg, Bucholz, and Mennell advised that chiefly the palm be used in the contact with the tissues. Hoffa and Mennell emphasized that the hand must fit the contour of the tissues. Hoffa specified different types of pétrissage, depending upon the parts of one or both hands that were used in performing the movement.

According to Ling and Murrell the motion is a rolling one,[37] the skin moving with the fingers, but Hoffa, Mitchell, Kellogg, Despard, Bucholz, and Mennell lifted the mass of tissues and made a squeezing movement. In addition to the rolling, Murrell added that the tissues are pressed and squeezed as one would squeeze out a sausage. Bucholz and Mennell advocated that the hand glide over the skin instead of the skin moving with the hand. Despard and Mennell alternately compressed the tissues between the thumb of one hand and the fingers of the other. Mezger lifted the tissues and kneaded them between the hands.[6] In addition to lifting the tissues for pétrissage, Despard also described a pétrissage in which the tissues are grasped and pressed down on the underlying structures and at the same time squeezed.

Murrell and Hoffa stated that the pressure is firm, Ling that it varies, and Mennell that it should be gentle. Mitchell and Despard alternately tightened and loosened the pressure. Kellogg stated that it must not be so great as to prevent deeper parts from gliding over still deeper structures.

Many authors mentioned that pétrissage is applied to muscle groups, individual muscles, or some part of a muscle. Ling mentioned specifically that the skin, subcutaneous tissues, and muscles are grasped,[37] while Mitchell was not specific; he mentioned only "tissues," and Murrell said "a portion of muscle or other tissue."

The direction is stated as centripetal by most authors; Hoffa and Mennell made compression transversely to the muscle fibers although the general movement was centripetal, and Bucholz stated that the succession of single manipulations might be either centripetal or centrifugal.

Kneading
(See Table III on page 24)

Only the most recent authors used kneading as a separate type of movement; the earlier ones used the French term pétrissage to describe the movement, which was very similar in many respects to the kneading described by the more recent users of massage.

Several authors described pétrissage as a kneading movement and made little differentiation between the two: other descriptions of kneading were very similar to those for pétrissage. Mennell stated that they very closely resemble each other, the only difference being that pétrissage is a picking-up movement with a lateral compression while in kneading the compression is vertical. Kellogg's concept is opposite to that of Mennell: he stated that the tissues are lifted in kneading and not in pétrissage. Graham stated that in kneading, the fingers and hand slip on the skin, while Kellogg stated definitely that the surface of the hand must not be allowed to slip along the surface of the skin.

Graham used kneading on the tissues beneath the skin, while Kellogg subdivided kneading, using "superficial" for skin and loose, cellular, underlying tissues and "deep" for muscles. Graham and Kellogg differed also on direction. Graham stated that it should be with the return circulation, and Kellogg stated that in "superficial" the relation to the veins is not important. Mennell began kneading of the limbs at the proximal portion of an area, progressing to the more distal. This kneading is performed with the two hands placed on opposite sides of the limbs, the whole palmar surfaces being in contact with the part. Gentle pressure is then performed, the hands usually working in opposite directions. He stated that the pressure is gentle, with alternating waves of compression and relaxation applied to a series of points, with the greatest pressure when the hand is engaged with the "lowest part of the circumference of the circle and least when at the opposite pole."

Friction
(See Table IV on pages 24 and 25)

From their descriptions of friction, there seems to be great confusion of concepts among the users of this form of massage. Kleen and Mennell differed from the other authors and used the plural "frictions," although they did not agree on pressure; Kleen stated that the pressure is quite hard and Mennell said it should be light, slowly progressing to deep, depending on the conditions present. Hoffa stated that the pressure seeks to penetrate deeply, Mitchell and Kellogg said that it is moderate.

Grosvenor and Graham stated that friction is given with long strokes, while most of the other authors stated that it is done with a small circular motion.[30] Graham said friction may be circular or rectilinear (the rectilinear movements may be parallel with or horizontal to the long axis of the limb). Kellogg stated that the direction is from "below upward," following the large veins, and the motion is centripetal, centrifugal, circular, or spiral rotary.[38] Kellogg also stated, and evidently Grosvenor and Graham agreed, that the hands should slip over the skin, and these authors used the entire palm of the hand. Hoffa, Bucholz, Despard, and Mennell stated that the movement is done with the ball of the thumb or fingers which keep contact with the skin and move it over the underlying tissues. Influenced by Ling,[37] several authors used the French term "massage à friction," which movement is no doubt similar to the contemporary "friction" or "frictions."

There is great variance in the tissues to which friction should be applied. Kleen, Mitchell, and Mennell used it on small areas, while Graham said each stroke extends from joint to joint. There seems to be two very distinct concepts in regard to this movement: one, that the friction occurs between the hand and the skin surface; the other (which seems to be more acceptable at the present), that the part of the hand being used is kept in contact with the skin, and the superficial tissues are moved over the deeper underlying ones.

Stroking and Effleurage
(See Tables V and VI on pages 26 and 27)

The descriptions of these movements are so similar that they may be discussed together. As in kneading and pétrissage, one finds continued use of the French and English terms, which are almost interchangeable. Mennell did not include the term "effleurage" in his classification of massage movements.

There is general agreement that the direction of the movement is centripetal. However, Mennell amd Kellogg differ. They both used the term "stroking," and Kellogg stated that the direction is "with the blood current in the arteries," although he did not mention the amount of pressure. Mennell divided stroking into "superficial" and "deep." Superficial stroking may be either centripetal or centrifugal, but the pressure, while firm, must be only the lightest touch possible to maintain contact. Deep stroking is in the direction of the venous and lymph flow.

Despard used both stroking and effleurage: the direction in both is centripetal, but the pressure in stroking is "vigorous" while in effleurage it "should vary according to the condition of the patient." Other factors in the movements were very similar, and she described the motion of effleurage as "stroking." Ling,[37] Mezger,[37] Kleen, and Mitchell also described the movement of effleurage as stroking.

Ling said the pressure in effleurage varies from the lightest touch to "one of considerable force." Murrell and Kleen said that it varies, while Hoffa and Bucholz used light pressure at the beginning of the stroke, increased it over the fleshy part of the muscle, and decreased it again at the end. Mitchell varied the pressure according to the region being treated and used heavy pressure on the upward stroke, keeping the hand in contact to return, but with much less pressure. Bucholz also kept the hand in contact for a return stroke, very lightly touching the skin.

Most authors agreed that stroking and effleurage are to be given over large areas. Mennell emphasized that the muscles must be relaxed, and Hoffa and Bucholz said that the movement should follow the anatomical outlines of the muscles.

Nearly all authors advocated the use of the palm of the hand for effleurage and stroking. In addition to the palm, some used the heel of the hand, its edge, the tips of the fingers, the ball of the thumb, and the "knuckles" for effleurage and stroking. Hoffa, Bucholz, Despard, and Mennell recommended that the palm should be in good contact and conform to the contour of the area being treated.

COMPONENTS OF MASSAGE
(See Table VII on pages 28 to 35)

The factors which must be considered as components in the application of massage techniques are: the direction of the movement: the amount of pressure; the rate and rhythm of the movements; the media used, including instruments other than the hand; the position of the patient and of the physical therapist; and the duration and frequency of the treatment.

Direction

Until the time of Hippocrates,[35] the literature shows that the direction of massage was centrifugal. The contribution of Hippocrates to medicine is outstanding, and he showed unusual genius in the use of massage as well as other methods of medical treatment. He advocated the centripetal direction for massage movements. He was unusual in his emphasis on clinical observation, and we can assume that his choice of direction was made from his clinical observations of the effect of the treatment. (The circulation of the blood was not discovered by Harvey until nearly two thousand years later.)

Asclepiades (125–56 B.C.),[35] a Roman who lived a few centuries later than Hippocrates, believed that the body was composed of regularly distributed canals in which nutritive juices moved. Sickness was a disturbance of the normal movement of these juices. He attempted to restore free movement of the nutritive juices by rubbing but gave no direction for the movement.

Galen, five centuries after Hippocrates, varied the direction of massage movements depending on the purpose of massage and its relation to exercise. Ling,[37] at the beginning of the nineteenth century, advocated a light stroking in the centrifugal direction, movements with deeper pressure in the centripetal. This concept has held through to the present-day writers. In the superficial stroking of Lucas-Championnière,[54] as followed by Mennell, the direction may be either centrifugal or centripetal but without deviation once the direction is established. These later writers were very definite in expressing the effects which are expected from the movements given in the centripetal direction as compared to those given in the centrifugal direction. Murrell advocated that the direction should be from below upwards and in the direction of the muscle fibers. Hoffa and Bucholz were among the first to mention that the direction should be with the venous and lymphatic circulation. Mennell said all deep movements of massage should be performed centripetally to aid the venous and lymphatic flow.

Many authors advocated beginning the movement at the proximal rather than the distal portion of a segment, but the direction of the pressure in each movement was in the direction of venous flow (centripetal) even though the succession of the movements was in the opposite (centrifugal) direction.

Pressure

Consideration of pressure seems to have been important from the earliest description of the massage movements, although there is great variance of opinions as to its application.

The Greek authors Herodikus (circa 500 B.C.) and Herodotus (484–425 B.C.) varied the pressure during the movement;[35] it was gentle at the first, then greater, and toward the end again gentle.

Later, Hippocrates differentiated the types of pressure, mentioning gentle, hard, soft, and moderate. He emphasized the importance of selection of pressure in technique in order to obtain a desired result. This is shown in the frequently quoted statement, "Hard rubbing binds; soft rubbing loosens; much rubbing causes parts to waste; moderate rubbing makes them grow."

Ambroise Paré,[30] the most renowned surgeon of the sixteenth century, recognized a difference in the amount of pressure used. He described three kinds of friction—gentle, medium, and vigrous—and the effects of each.

In the fifteenth, sixteenth, seventeenth, and beginning of the eighteenth centuries, there seemed to be growing emphasis placed upon heavy pressure, the extremist being Admiral Henry (1731–1823),[35] of the British Navy who believed that "great violence" was important. He described some of the manipulations as being painful, "but they cease to be so if persevered in, and become even pleasant." Beveridge emphasized the importance of touch in varying pressure and the difference in the effect produced depending upon the amount of pressure. In the early part of the nineteenth century, he wrote, "The finger of a good rubber will descend upon an excited and painful nerve as gently as the dew on the grass, but upon a torpid callosity as heavily as the hoof of an elephant."

Mezger varied the pressure with the type of movement;[6] that for effleurage was gentle and for "massage à friction" was "with considerable force." This force must have been considerable as Colombo,[11] one of his contemporaries, stated that Mezger's patients frequently had blue spots on their bodies. Zabludowski, who was known as the "king of German masseurs," criticized the gentle massage advocated by Lucas-Championnière for the treatment of fractures. Zabludowski said that when massage became painless, it ceased to be massage and was merely treatment by suggestion. However, in his book written later (1903), Zabludowski wrote that massage is not painful in most cases and when it becomes necessarily painful, the pain should subside. Bucholz, writing in 1917, did not agree with Zabludowski's early concepts. He believed all needed effects could be obtained without such abuse of force.

At about this same time, Kleen and Hoffa showed they appreciated the finesse of technique, together with knowledge, and they regulated the pressure according to the bulk of the tissues, increasing it when working on the belly of a muscle and lessening it at the ends of the muscle. (In this we see recognition of the early concepts of Herodikus and Herodotus.) They also stated that the proper amount can be judged only by practice.

Throughout the late nineteenth and early twentieth centuries, many authors gave the impression that the greater the pressure, the more effective is the massage. They began the treatment or series of treatments with gentle pressure and "worked up" the tolerance of the patient to greater pressure. Kellogg stated that the patient's tolerance is established by prolonged treatment, beginning gently and gradually increasing until almost the "whole strength of the operator might be employed without injuring the patient." Despard stated that the "vigour" and amount of pressure should vary according to the condition of the patient, being always gentle at the beginning of the course of treatment and gradually increasing as the patient improves.

Mennell was outstanding in his rationale for the use of massage. Of pressure he stated that the amount is dependent solely upon the relaxation of the musculature. When the muscles are relaxed throughout the treatment, even a light pressure must influence every structure throughout the part being treated. He believed the movement may be "deep" without in any sense being forcible. His reasoning was that if the muscles are relaxed they offer no more resistance to the movement than so much fluid, and any pressure applied on the surface will be transmitted freely to all structures under the hand. He said that practice with a skill that is born only of a delicate sense of touch will show how very light may be the pressure which will suffice to compress any structure to its fullest extent and, therefore, incidentally to empty the veins and lymphatic spaces. He also said, "The delusion is deep rooted—and will die hard—that 'stimulation' in massage is impossible without the expenditure of muscle energy and vigour. A delusion, nevertheless, it is."

Rate and Rhythm

Some authors vaguely mentioned the rate of massage movements, but few made statements regarding rhythm. Others combined the two.

Of the early writers,[35] Herodikus and Herodotus both associated pressure and rate, gentle and slow in the beginning, rapid and heavy in the interim, and ending slow and gentle. Hippocrates, in describing treatment of a dislocated shoulder, stated "it is necessary to rub the shoulder gently and smoothly." None of the users of massage after Hippocrates made mention of rate or rhythm until the eighteenth and nineteenth centuries. Beveridge evidently considered great speed an advantage, for he stated that flexibility of the fingers is important as it permits rapidity of motion. Ling varied rate according to the type of movement: effleurage should be given slowly; rolling, shaking, and tapotement rapidly. Mezger agreed that effleurage should be given slowly.

Graham, Kellogg, and Bucholz were specific in the number of strokes to be given per minute but were not definite as to the distance which is covered in each stroke; therefore the number of strokes had no specific relationship to rate. These authors differed in the number of strokes they specified. For friction, Graham specified 90 to 180 per minute. Bucholz stated that speed depends on the effect desired. ("In irritable cases a slow gentle stroke may produce a marked effect, while in treating an atrophic limb of an otherwise healthy person, considerable speed, up to 50 to 60 times a minute or more, with a good deal of pressure may be applied.") However, Kellogg stated that it depends on the type of movement and stated the distance to be covered. Stroking, he specified, should not be more than one or two inches per second; friction 30 to 80 strokes per minute, varying with the length of stroke; and pétrissage "not too rapid," 30 to 90 per minute, "more rapid in small parts."

Kleen varied the rate with the area treated: effleurage on the shoulder and back he thought should be rapid. Lucas-Championnière emphasized that massage should be slow and uniform, a rhythmical repetition.[54] Zabludowski stated that the area covered determines the speed to some extent, compared rhythm to that of music, and suggested that a metronome be used in practice, but not as a regular guide. Despard varied the rate and rhythm according to the effect desired. She said that for a soothing effect effleurage should be given slowly and rhythmically, and for a stimulating effect the strokes should be "quick and strong." The rate and vigor, she stated, should vary according to the condition of the patient, and all movements should be performed rhythmically.

In stroking movements some authors distinguished between the rate of the primary stroke and the return stroke, making the return stroke more rapid, which makes an uneven rhythm. Mitchell advised this and also stated that one of the common faults of massage is to give the movements too fast. Mennell said the essentials of superficial stroking are that the movements must be slow, gentle, and rhythmical, and there must be no hesitancy or irregularity about it; the time between the end of the stroke and the beginning of the next should be identical with the time of stroking throughout the movement. He believed the rhythm must be even in order to produce an even stimulus. As a rate for the stroke from shoulder to hand, he gave 15 movements per minute. In deep stroking, he said, there is no need for great rapidity as the flow of blood in the veins is slow and of the lymph channels even slower. He stated of kneading that excessive rapidity is inimical to success, and that in "frictions" the rhythm should be slow and unbroken.

Media

The writings of Homer imply that, as early as 1000 B.C., an oily medium was used for massage. According to Homer's *Odyssey,* beautiful women rubbed and anointed the war-worn heroes to rest and refresh them. Herodotus advised that a "greasy mixture" should be poured over the body before rubbing, and Plato (427–347 B.C.)[30] and Socrates (470–399 B.C.)[30] refer to the benefit received from anointing with oils and rubbing as an "assuager of pain." Olive oil was used, and it was believed that the oil itself had some curative value. Roman history records that Cicero received great improvement in his health from his anointer.

Celsus made a distinction between rubbing and unction or anointing.[30, 35] The rubbing in of greasy substances he called unction. Other authors later contended that unction could not be performed without friction of some sort. In the days of Galen, the massage following exercise was applied with a greater amount of oil than that given before exercise. He recommended rubbing with a towel to produce redness followed by rubbing with oil for the purpose of ''warming up'' and softening the body previous to exercise.

Henry was unique in the media which he used.[30, 35] He devised various instruments and tools which he said ''would prevent the nerves and tendons from falling asleep or getting fixed'' and, by keeping these structures in constant action, ''the blood would pass quickly through the blood vessels, leaving no fur behind it, so that ossification which so frequently terminates the human existence is prevented.'' The instruments were made of wood and bone; the knobs were preserved, and others were made by the use of a file. Ribs of cattle were used principally, as it was of great advantage to have them bent. He also used a hammer with a piece of cork covered with leather as well as the rounded end of a glass vial. Graham followed a similar method to a certain extent in percussion. He suggested that the back of a brush or the sole of a slipper could be used but even better were India rubber balls attached to steel or whalebone handles.

In exceptional circumstances, Murrell said, a bundle of swan's feathers, lightly tied together, could be used for tapotement. Kellogg used the fingernail, the end of a lead pencil, a wooden toothpick, or the head of a pin for reflex stroking. On the island of Tonga in the early nineteenth century it is reported that ''three or four little children tread under their feet the whole body of the patient.''[30] At about this same time, the Russians and Finns used a bundle of birch twigs for flagellation preceding steam baths, and the Hawaiians gave massage under water.

The more recent users of massage differ in opinion regarding the use of a medium for massage. Some object to any sort of medium, and those who use a medium choose either an oily lubricant of some sort or a powder. Some of the reasons given for ''no medium'' or ''dry massage'' are: it is cleaner; it gives a more certain feeling to the hand; the movements are steadier; it is more stimulating in effect; it is unnecessary to expose the patient's body. It seems incredible, but massage frequently has been given over the patient's clothing. Galen records that when a gymnast inquired of Quintas what was the value of anointment (rubbing with oil), he replied, ''It makes you take off your tunic.''

Many substances are suggested by those who use oily lubricants; both liquid and solid lubricants are used. The more commonly mentioned are: olive oil, glycerine, coconut oil, oil of sweet almonds, and neat's-foot oil. Some users prefer solid lubricants because the flowing oils are ''hard to handle.'' The solid lubricants suggested are fat, wool fat, petroleum jelly, lanolin, hog's lard, cold cream, and cocoa butter. Zabludowski was quite specific in his preference for white Virginia petroleum jelly because it was ''odorless and tasteless and quite neutral.'' He said that the chief basis for the use of any lubricant comes from clinical experience and not from any real scientific experiment. The advantages listed by those who recommend oily lubricants are: they make the skin soft, smooth, and slippery; prevent the pain of pulling hair; and prevent acne. Some of those who oppose the use of oily lubricants claim that they promote the growth of hair.

Others who use a medium recommend the use of a powder, as they believe it is more pleasant for general massage, makes deep kneading possible, and improves the sense of touch. Several users recommend its use particularly to prevent the moisture of the masseur's hands from causing an abrasion on the patient's skin. Grosvenor recommended the use of ''fine hair powder'' and writers of more recent date suggest talcum or boric acid powder. A few writers suggest soapsuds as a medium.

Mennell said the selection of a medium is a personal factor and believed the best is the simplest namely: French chalk, which might be improved by adding oil. He, as well as other users, recommended an oily medium, especially when the skin is dry and scaly. Some suggested its use on children, the aged, and emaciated individuals. Of the later users in this group the reason, although not so stated, undoubtedly was to avoid abrasion of sensitive skin, as contrasted to the belief of the early writers that the medium itself had a curative value.

Position of Patient and Physical Therapist

The early writers gave very little indication of the position of the patient or of the masseur while giving massage. There is no written information of this until about the seventeenth century. However, a bas-relief showing massage for the returned soldiers, as described in Homer's *Odyssey,* depicts massage given to Ulysses on his return from war. He is seated and the masseuse is in a most uncomfortable crouching position in front of him giving massage to his leg. Alpinus said the patient should be "extended horizontally." Many of the later writers gave the positions quite in detail and emphasized that the patient should be relaxed (this, after they placed the patient in such a position that relaxation would seem to be utterly impossible). Very few of them stated reasons for the position to be assumed and they seemed to disregard entirely any influence which gravity might have upon the venous and lymphatic flow. Ling emphasized that the muscles must be relaxed for many movements and yet described rolling and shaking of the arm with the patient seated, holding the arm in a horizontal position, with the hand on the table or back of a chair.[37]

Grosvenor's position for massage of the lower extremity, as described by Cleoburey, is: "The female rubber (for Mr. Grosvenor always employed females) [is] seated on a low stool, and taking the patient's limb in her lap (which position gave her command over it) so as to enable her to rub with extended hands." The position of the patient is not stated. One would assume that he or she was seated in a position similar to that of Ulysees as shown in the Greek bas-relief referred to previously.

Graham said the patient should be in a comfortable position, with joints midway between flexion and extension, and warned that if the "manipulator" was too close to the patient he would be cramped in his movements, and that if he was too far away the movements would be indefinite, superficial, and lacking in energy.

Kleen described a bench on which the patient was to lie and which was approachable from all sides, the masseur standing or sitting beside it. He gave much detail for positions of the patient for treatment of various areas. For massage of the neck and throat he had the patient sit on the bench.

Hoffa recommended support to the entire length of the part of the body which is being treated so that the muscles are relaxed, yet he had the patient sit on a stool for massage of the head, neck, shoulder, and upper arm. For massage of the elbow, forearm, hand, and fingers, an illustration shows the patient sitting with these parts resting on a table. For the leg and foot, the patient sits on the table with the foot supported in the lap of the masseur. He said that the masseur's position should be "comfortable and not strained," always beside the patient's bed, and avoiding as much as possible frequent and unnecessary change of position. For the thigh, the patient is lying and the masseur sits beside him.

Zabludowski recommended a comfortable and relaxed position for the patient. The position depended upon the part treated. The patient's glasses were to be removed and the lighting and room temperature adjusted to insure his comfort. He stated that some work might even be done with the patient in the standing position or that small children might be held in the lap if a table was not available. He emphasized the posture of the masseur and said the standing position was preferred. The masseur should have a sure footing and a coordinated movement to ease his work and eliminate much flexing and extending in many joints. Zabludowski added some interesting rules for the masseur: he should watch his watch chain so it does not bother the patient; he should wear glasses instead of "pince-nez" which might slide off his nose if he perspired; he should wear a jersey (knit) undershirt, heavy or light according to the season; he should not work in street clothes, should remove his rings, have short sleeves and even remove things in his pockets that are in the way when he is sitting.

Mitchell recommended that the patient should be reclining and for some areas that the "operator" sit on the edge of the bed with the patient's foot in his lap. Bucholz said the patient should be in a comfortable position, one which would also allow the "operator" to work with sufficient comfort. He did not favor the sitting position for massaging the legs, although he stated it might be used for the foot and calf if the patient was sitting on a table and the "operator" in front of him on a chair.

Despard recommended that the patient should be in a comfortable position and the muscles relaxed; yet for back stroking she said the patient might be standing with hands resting against the wall or other support.

Mennell said the points that require most attention in performing all stroking movements are the positions of the patient and of the masseur, and the relative position of one to the other. He gave no set rules for positions of either, but said there should be a reason for every position of the masseur and for the position in which the part under treatment is placed. Some of the illustrations in his text show the masseur in the standing and in the sitting position. He used an illustration of stroking of the lower extremity to point out some of the common faults of positons of the patient and of the masseur.

In discussing the effect of massage on the venous flow, he considered the effect of gravity of great importance and recommended that the patient be recumbent on the table in a position which allows relaxation of abdominal muscles with the thighs supported in order to assist in the venous and lymphatic flow from the distal part of the lower extremity. In the treatment of edema of an extremity, he recommended elevation of the part while giving the massage.

Duration

Galen was one of the first users of massage to mention the duration of a treatment. He used the trial and error method. He wrote, "What shall be the duration of the rubbing it is impossible to declare in words; but the director, being experienced in these matters, on the first day must form a conjecture, which shall not be very accurate, but the next day, having already acquired some experience in the constitution of this subject, he will reduce his conjecture continually to greater accuracy."

Grosvenor[18, 35] was very specific in his directions for the duration of treatment. He said that friction should be at first continued for one hour, "observing always to rub by the watch."

Murrell said the entire time of a local massage should not exceed eight to ten minutes and that other authorities thought four minutes was enough.

Kleen believed the duration of a treatment was important but that no hard and fast rule could be given. Local massage, he thought, usually should last fifteen minutes and general massage at least half an hour and sometimes longer, while Hoffa suggested ten to twenty minutes for local and thirty to forty-five minutes for general massage. Zabludowski said the duration may be from five to thirty minutes depending on the affected area (its size), age of the patient, duration of illness, constitution of the patient, and habits of the patient. He gave an estimate of the entire length of time which the treatment should be continued, which he said is dependent upon the condition to be treated, the prognosis, and so forth, but which usually is from two to three weeks.

According to Graham, the condition of the patient and the effect of the massage should determine the duration of the treatment. Bucholz said the duration of the treatment should depend upon the effect desired. In fresh injury he stated that five to ten minutes may be adequate, while a general massage should be forty to fifty minutes.

Despard gave a definite period of time for each area of the body and said the duration of the treatment should increase as the condition of the patient improves.

Mennell believed it is necessary to consider the age of the patient when administering massage, particularly when the aim is solely to secure a reflex effect. In the young and the aged the duration of treatment should be lessened. In the treatment of neurasthenia, Mennell said the maximum duration is seventy-five minutes, which may be attained in comparatively few cases and never during the earlier stages of treatment. At first, twenty minutes is often sufficient and may be gradually increased and toward the end should be decreased in a similar manner. In cases of injury, however, he emphasized the danger of prolonging the series of the massage treatments in lieu of active exercise as the patient improves.

Frequency

Celsus, who was not a physician, was a noted medical author, and in his *De Medicina* he wrote merely as an encyclopedist, presenting the ideas from the available literature which appealed to him.[35] We may presume, therefore, that his writings express some of the ideas which were popular at that time. He gave some details of massage techinque and appreciated the value of correct dosage. He stated that "we should pay no attention to those who define numerically how often anyone is to be rubbed; for this must be gathered from the individual; and if he is very feeble, fifty times may be enough; if more robust, it may be requisite to rub two hundred times, and between both limits according to the strength." He also believed it should be done less frequently in the case of a woman than a man and less frequently for a child or old person than a young man.

Grosvenor advised daily treatment (more or less as the case would permit) and gradually increased to three times daily.[18, 35] Murrell also believed in frequent treatment, three or four times daily, but the length of his treatments were much shorter than those of Grosvenor.

Kleen believed massage should be at least once daily and in some cases of injury several times daily. Hoffa advised daily massage. Zabludowski advocated daily massage in most cases but advised that the physical and psychological reactions of the patient should determine the frequency. If quick results are desired, he believed treatments should be given twice daily, but in cases which necessitated a "weaning from massage" the frequency should be gradually lessened to two or three treatments per week.

Graham recognized the frequency of treatment as a part of the dosage of massage which should be regulated according to the condition of the patient. He associated force with the frequency and duration of treatment, local massage being done frequently and general massage at least once daily. As contrasted to Zabludowski's weaning from massage, Graham said the frequency may be increased after four or five treatments.

Bucholz said that the frequency of treatment will depend largely on the patient's social condition but advised twice daily in many surgical cases. He believed it to be wise to begin with short sessions and increase according to the patient's reaction.

In the components of massage technique as recommended by many of these authorities, there seems to be no physiological basis for their technique, particularly in relation to pressure, rate of movement, and the positioning of the patient. The heavy pressure advocated in the fifteenth, sixteenth, seventeenth, and early eighteenth centuries was supplanted by more gentle massage as introduced by Lucas-Championnière[54] and Mennell in the early twentieth century; yet one is astonished that to a certain extent this was appreciated by Hippocrates,[35] who certainly did not have the scientific physiological information that is available today. Bucholz and Hoffa at the beginning of the twentieth century began to show some rational application of massage technique based upon a knowledge of physiology, but in this respect Mennell is outstanding and is the most rational of all.

TABLE I. *Terminology of Massage*

Date	Name	Place	Terminology
		Circa 1000 B.C. to 500 A.D.	
1000 B.C.	Homeric Age		Anointing Rubbing
Circa 500 B.C.	Herodikus	Greece	Rubbing Friction
484–425 B.C.	Herodotus	Greece	Rubbing Friction
460–380 B.C.	Hippocrates	Greece	Rubbing Anatripsis
128–56 B.C.	Asclepiades	Rome	Friction
25 B.C.–50 A.D.	Celsus, Aurelius	Rome	Friction Rubbing Unction
130–200 A.D.	Galen, Claudius	Rome	Tripsis Anatripsis Tripsisparaskeulasthke Apotherapeia
325–403 A.D.	Oribasius	Rome	Apotherapeia 1. Bathing 2. Friction 3. Inunction

Other terms used in this period were pommeling, squeezing, and pinching.

TABLE I. *Terminology of Massage—Continued*

Date	Name	Place	Terminology
		15th, 16th, 17th Centuries	
1492-1541	Paracelsus	Switzerland	Friction
1510-1590	Paré, Ambroise	France	Friction
1553-1617	Alpinus, Prospero	Italy	Rubbing Maxalation Manipulations Pressure
1537-1619	Fabricius, Hieronymus	Italy	Rubbing Kneading
1624-1689	Sydenham, Thomas	England	Friction
1660-1742	Hoffmann, Friedrich	Prussia	Apotherapeia

"Sau-Tsai-Tow-Hooe," published in Japan in the 16th century, shows that the terms pressure, percussion, and vibration (and rubbing) were in use by the Japanese from very early periods. "Cong-Fou of the Tao-Sse" is the Chinese expression used to apply to physicians who use mechanical therapeutics. They rubbed the entire body with the hands and gently pressed the muscles between the fingers.

18th and 19th Centuries

Dates	Name	Country	Terms
1731–1823	Henry, Admiral		Rubbing
1742–1823	Grosvenor, John	England	Friction
1774–1839	Beveridge, William	Scotland	Finger rubbing
1776–1839	Ling, Peter H.	Sweden	Effleurage Petrissage Massage a friction Rolling Slapping Pinching Shaking Vibration Tapotement Joint movement
1819 (date of writing)	Balfour, William	Scotland (Edinburgh)	Compression Percussion Friction

1839–1901 (1909)	Mezger, Johann Georg	Holland (Amsterdam)	Effleurage
			Massage a friction
			Petrissage
			Tapotement
			  1. Beating
			  2. Clapping

19th and 20th Centuries

Dates	Name	Country	Terms
1843–1913	Lucas-Championnière, Just Marie	France	Glucokinesis Effrayante

TABLE I. *Terminology of Massage* — Continued

Date	Name	Place	Terminology

1847-1923	Kleen, Emil Andreas Gabriel	Sweden	Effleurage-stroking
			Frictions-rubbing
			Pétrissage
			  1. Pinching
			  2. Rolling
			  3. Kneading
			Tapotement
			  1. Slapping
			  2. Pushing
			  3. Beating
			  4. Clapping
			  5. Vibration
			  6. Shaking

1848-1928	Graham, Douglas	United States	Friction Kneading Manipulation Rolling Pinching Percussion Movement Maxalation Pressure Squeezing

1851-1906	Zabludowski, J.B.	Germany	Pressure manipulations
			  1. Intermittent pounding
			  2. Slapping
			  3. Vibration
			  4. Hacking
			  5. Pinching
			  6. Shaking
			Stroking manipulations
			  1. Rubbing
			  2. Kneading
			  3. Muscle rolling
			  4. Pressing
			  5. Stroking

The terms used by islanders of Tonga at this time were Toogi-Toogi, Mili, and Fota. That of the Hawaiians was Lomi-Lomi.

Dates	Name	Country	Techniques

1852-1943	Kellogg, J. H.	United States	Describes 37 movements including:
			Touch
			Stroking
			Friction
			Pétrissage
			Kneading
			  1. Superficial
			  2. Deep
			    a. Palmar kneading
			    b. Fist kneading
			    c. Digital kneading
			    d. Rolling
			    e. Wringing
			    f. Chucking
			Vibration
			Percussion
			Joint movement

1853-1912	Murrell, William	Scotland and England	Effleurage Petrissage Friction Massage à friction Tapotement

1859-1907	Hoffa, Albert	Germany	Effleurage
			Stroking
			Friction
			Finger friction
			Pétrissage
			  1. Two-hand
			  2. Two-finger
			Vibration
			Tapotement
			  1. Hacking
			  2. Slapping

1859-1917	Mitchell, John K.	United States (Philadelphia)	Effleurage
			Pétrissage
			  1. Rolling
			  2. Fist kneading
			  3. Digital kneading
			  4. Wringing
			  5. Pulling
			Friction
			Tapotement

TABLE I. *Terminology of Massage* — Continued

Date	Name	Place	Terminology

1874-
(book published in 1917)
	Bucholz, C. Herman	United States	Rubbing
			  1. Simple
			  2. Effleurage
			  3. Stroking
			Kneading
			  1. Petrissage
			    a. Deep
			    b. Grasping
			    c. Lifting
			    d. Wringing
			    e. Pressing
			    f. Rolling
			    g. Harping
			  2. Friction
			Clapping
			Shaking
			Tapotement

1880-1957	Mennell, James B.	England	Stroking
			  1. Deep
			  2. Superficial
			Compression
			  1. Kneading
			  2. Pétrissage
			  3. Frictions
			  4. Pressure
			Percussion
			  1. Hacking
			  2. Clapping
			  3. Beating
			  4. Vibration
			  5. Shaking

Books published
in 1910 and 1932
	Despard, Louisa L.	England	Effleurage
			  1. Deep
			  2. Superficial
			Stroking
			Massage a friction
			Pétrissage
			Tapotement
			  1. Clapping
			  2. Hacking
			  3. Beating
			  4. Pounding
			Vibration
			Shaking

Books published in 1944 and 1952	Dicke, Elizabeth	Germany	Stroking 1. Pulling 2. Pull and hook-on 3. Widening
Book published in 1959	Cyriax, James	England	Deep massage Deep friction
Book published in 1961	Tappan, Frances	United States	Effleurage Petrissage Tapotement Friction Vibration
Book published in 1962	Ebner, Maria	England	Lifting Pressure Stroking Tensile stroke Lifting stroke Stretching

TABLE II. *Description of Massage Movements: Pétrissage*

Name	Direction	Pressure	Part of Hand	Motion	Tissues
Ling		Varying.	Grasped between thumb and fingers.	Kneading movement. Rolled between thumb and fingers. Skin moves with fingers.	Skin, subcutaneous tissue, and muscle.
Mezger				Lifting, then kneading between the hands.	Some part of muscle.
Murrell	Centripetal. Hands move simultaneously in opposite directions.	Firm.	Both hands or fingers of one hand. Thumb and fingers wide apart.	Pressed and rolled between fingers and subadjacent tissues. Skin must move with hands. Squeeze as one would squeeze out a sausage.	Portion of muscle or other tissue.
Kleen				Rollings, kneadings, or pinchings.	
Hoffa (one hand)		Not with finger tips, but chiefly with base of thumb and index finger.	Chiefly base of thumb and index finger – not tips.	Lift from underlying tissues. Press out like sponge.	Grasp entire bulk of muscle. Begin at insertion.
(two hand)	Transversely to muscle fibers backward and forward in opposite directions.		Both hands.	Pick up and squeeze out.	Crosswise before masseur. Around as much of muscle as possible.
(two finger)		Firm.	Tip of thumb, index, and middle finger.	Twisting movement of the skin.	Muscles which spread out and cannot be grasped by entire hand and particularly if covered by fascia.
Mitchell		Close – alternately tightening and loosening of the hold.	Whole palm and parts of fingers nearest palm – not finger tips. Fingers close together.	Lifting mass a little. Kneading skin to move with hands over underlying tissues.	"Tissues."
Kellogg	Upward.	Not so great as to prevent deeper parts from gliding over still deeper structures.	As much of palmar surface as possible. Fingers close together and opposing the thenar eminence.	Tissues squeezed and lifted from bone or deeper tissues, rolled, and stretched. Grasp released when strain is at its maximum.	Individual muscles or muscle groups.

Despard	Centripetal.	Intermittent.	One or both hands.	Grasped, raised from attachment (picked up, lifted from underlying tissues), then compressed alternately between fingers of one hand and thumb of other. Move onward between each compression. or Grasped, the tissues pressed down upon underlying structures and at same time squeezed.	Muscles, singly or in groups.
Bucholz	Follows outline of muscle. Succession of single manipulations may be either centripetal or centrifugal.		One or both working simultaneously. As much of hand as possible held close to skin.	Grasped, lifted as much as possible from base, and kneaded or wrung. Glided 1 or 2 inches, repeated from one end of muscle to the other. If muscle cannot be lifted, rolled and pressed.	Muscles or muscle groups.
Mennell	Compression lateral.	Gentle.	Entire surface of hand relaxed.	Entire muscle group picked up in hands and squeezed, compressing alternately between thumb of one hand and fingers of the other. Hands glided gently over surface.	Muscles.

TABLE III.   Description of Massage Movements: Kneading

Name	Direction	Pressure	Part of Hand	Motion	Tissues
Graham	From insertion to origin of the muscles, with return circulation.		As much as possible of fingers and hand. Slip on skin.	Kneading, rolling, squeezing, manipulatory. Circulatory.	Tissues beneath skin.
Kellogg (superficial)	Relation to veins not important.		Thumb and last two phalanges of first or first and second fingers.	Essentially a pinching movement. Skin simultaneously compressed and lifted from underlying bone or muscle.	Skin and loose cellular tissues underlying.
(deep)		Little on thin tissues, greater on thick firm tissues.	Surface of hand not allowed to slip along surface of skin.	Grasped or compressed.	Muscles.
(digital)			Ends of fingers and thumbs alone.	Tissues rubbed and pressed against underlying bony surface.	
Mennell	Centripetal. Begin proximal portion, advance to more distal. Compression vertical.	Gentle; alternating wave of compression and relaxation; applied to a series of points, with greatest pressure when hand is engaged with lowest part of circle; least pressure when at opposite pole.	Whole of palmar surface of both hands on opposite sides of limb, alternating heel of hand and then fingers.	Circular, hands working in opposite directions.	Muscle mass.

TABLE IV.   Description of Massage Movements: Friction

Name	Direction	Pressure	Part of Hand	Motion	Tissues
Grosvenor	One hand ascends as other descends.		Palm of hand.	Long strokes.	
Kleen (frictions)		Quite hard.	Volar side of thumb or three middle fingers or sometimes the base of the hand, occasionally with entire hand flat.	Rubbings.	Small surface.
Hoffa	Circular.	Seeks to penetrate deeply.	Tips of fingers, either thumb or middle and index finger.	Index and middle fingers seek firm point of support. Ball of thumb held stiffly. Little circular movements. Thumb moves with skin.	Part placed on solid support.

Graham	Circular or rectilinear. Latter may be vertical or parallel to long axis of the limb; or horizontal, transverse or at right angles to the long axis.	Upward strokes, stronger returning lightly, graze surface for soothing influence. Heavy in centripetal direction.		Both hands move at same time; one ascends as other descends.	Each stroke reaching from joint to joint.
Mitchell		Moderate — steady.	Thumb or finger tips of one or more fingers. Hand to slip over surface.	Rubbing in small circles.	Areas where larger grasp of petrissage is not possible.
Kellogg	From below upward, following large veins. Centripetal, centrifugal, circular, spiral rotary.	Considerable, depending on area; amount never such that the hand will not slip over surface or so great as to interfere with arterial circulation.	Hand.	Slipping over skin.	
Bucholz	Circular.			Moving skin over underlying parts.	
Mennell (frictions)	Circular or transversely to long axis of muscle fibers.	Light — slowly progressive to deep, depending on condition present.	Usually tips of fingers or tip or ball of thumb.		Muscles must be relaxed.
Despard	Circular.		Palmar aspects or tips of fingers or ball of thumb, also dorsal aspect of middle phalanges of fingers.	Moving tissues upon underlying ones.	Tissues.

TABLE V. *Description of Massage Movements: Effleurage*

Name	Direction	Pressure	Part of Hand	Motion	Tissues
Ling	Centripetal.	Varying from lightest touch to "one of considerable force."		Stroking.	
Mezger	Centripetal.	Superficial and gentle.	Flat.	Stroking.	
Murrell	Direction of muscle fibers, centripetally.	Varying.	Palm or knuckles.		
Kleen	Centripetal.	Varying.	Large portion with hand flat, its ulnar or radial side or with thumb and forefinger. One or both hands.	Strokings.	Large area of skin.
Hoffa	Toward the heart.	Begin lightly; then increase and diminish again toward end of stroke.	Conform to part treated as broadly and closely as possible. Whole of hand or part of it (according to extent of part treated) flat for broad surfaces; ball of thumb; finger tip; knuckle (when part is covered by thick fascia).	Hand conforms closely to limb; thumb and finger tips proceed along grooves between muscles.	Follows strictly anatomic structures of muscles along grooves between muscles, over veins and lymph channels. Begins beyond affected part, extends over affected region, finishes in well part.
Mitchell	Centripetal.	Depends on region. Return stroke much less pressure than upward but keeping contact.	Flat hand, heel of hand, edge of hand, thumb, thumb and fingers or finger tips.	Stroking.	
Bucholz	Centripetal. With lymphatic flow.	Slight at distal part of muscle, increase over fleshy part, decrease toward proximal part. Return stroke in centrifugal direction, touching skin lightly.	Fits as closely as possible to muscle.	Where possible, lift up and grasp around muscle and stroke with thumb and fingers. If not possible to lift, hand presses muscle against underlying base.	Anatomical outlines of muscles.
Despard	Centripetal.	Vary according to condition of patient.	Whole of one or both hands or palmar surface of fingers, and thumb. Hand molded to fit part.	Stroking.	

TABLE VI. *Description of Massage Movements: Stroking*

Name	Direction	Pressure	Part of Hand	Motion	Tissues
Kellogg	"Blood current in arteries."		Fingers, palm, knuckles.	Touch combined with motion.	
Mennell (super- ficial)	Centripetal or centrifugal, but continue same direction is established.	Superficial — firm but lightest touch.	Flat surface. Hand supple to mould to contour of limb and —perfect contact with wide area.	Rhythmical	Extended area of body. Muscles must be relaxed.
(deep)	Centripetal with venous and lymph flow.	Deep — light.			
Despard	Centripetal.	Vigorous.	Tips of fingers.		

TABLE VII. *Components of Massage Techniques*

Name	Direction	Pressure	Rate and Rhythm	Medium	Position of Patient and Physical Therapist	Duration	Frequency
			Circa 500 B.C. to 500 A.D.				
Herodikus (circa 500 B.C.)	Centrifugal.	Initial – gentle; interim – heavy; end – gentle.	Slow beginning; rapid interim; slow ending.	Greasy mixture.			
Herodotus (484-425 B.C.)	Centrifugal.	Initial – gentle; interim – heavy; end – gentle.	Slow beginning; rapid interim; slow ending.				
Hippocrates (460-380 B.C.)	Centripetal.	"Gently" – hard rubbing, soft rubbing, moderate rubbing.	Smooth.			Much – or moderate	
Asclepiades (128-56 B.C.)		Gentle.					
Celsus (25 B.C.-50 A.D.)				Greasy substances.		Regulated entirely by strength and reaction of patient. Total of 50 to 200 times.	
Galen (130-200 A.D.)	Tripsis – centripetal; anatripsis – centrifugal.			Towel for tripsis; olive oil – greater amount for apotherapeia.			
			15th, 16th, 17th Centuries				
Paracelsus (1492-1541)		Friction – gentle, medium, vigorous.					
Paré (1517-1590)		Friction – gentle, medium, vigorous.					
Alpinus (1553-1617)					Patient extended horizontally.		

18th and 19th Centuries

Name						
Henry (1731–1823)			Tools of wood and bone, hammer and piece of cork covered with leather, rounded end of glass vial.	Great violence important.		
Beveridge (1774–1839)	Lightest touch to extremely heavy pressure.	Great speed.				
Ling (1776–1839)	Effleurage — centrifugal or centripetal. / Effleurage — lightest touch to considerable force. Pétrissage — carries throughout the movement.	Rolling, shaking and tapotement rapid. Some movement, slowly.	Oil.	Muscles relaxed, Arm extended horizontally, hand supported on table or back of chair.	Tapotement – short.	
Kellgren			Dry massage.			
Balfour (1819 — date of writing)	Deep rubbing; firm compression.					
Grosvenor (1742–1823)	Friction — one hand ascends while other descends.		Fine hair powder.	"Rubber" seated on stool with patient's limb in her lap, "which position gave her control."	Friction 1 hour, gradually increased to dosage of 1 hour 3 times a day, "observing always to rub by the watch."	Maximum three times a day.

TABLE VII. Components of Massage Techniques—Continued

Name	Direction	Pressure	Rate and Rhythm	Medium	Position of Patient and Physical Therapist	Duration	Frequency
Mezger (1853–1901 [1909])	Effleurage — centripetal; massage a friction — circular and centripetal.	Effleurage — superficial and gentle; massage a friction—considerable force.	Effleurage — slow.	Fat well rubbed into skin.			
Graham (1848–1928)	In general, centripetal from extremities to trunk with return circulation from insertion to origin. Friction—circular, heavy pressure of strokes centripetal; circular and rectilinear parallel to long axis of limbs or horizontal transverse or at right angles to long axis.		Friction — 90-180 per minute.	Back of brush, sole of slipper. India rubber balls attached to whalebone handle for percussion.	Comfortable position with joints midway between flexion and extension. If "manipulator" is too near the patient, he will be cramped; if too far away, his movements will be indefinite, superficial, and lacking in energy.	Local, not more than 8-10 minutes.	Short sittings frequently repeated 3 or 4 times daily.
Murreil (1853–1912)	Pétrissage — hand simultaneously opposite directions from below upwards. Effleurage — follow direction of muscle fibers.	Pétrissage — firm pressure.	Rate varies — initial and final quick; massage a friction, quick; effleurage, varying.	Dry massage. Bundle of swan's feathers may be used for tapotement.		Based on effect on patient and frequency of manipulation.	Regulates dosage.
Kleen (1847–1923)	Effleurage of limbs — centripetal; of abdomen — circular; throat — from top downward.	Quite hard pressure — amount can be judged only by practice. Pétrissage — firm over belly of muscle; new patient and painful cases, begin with little force, gradually increased.	Effleurage — should be rapid. Stroking on back — rapid.	Glycerine, petrolatum, lanolin, lard, cold cream, olive oil, coconut oil, talcum and other powders. Lard preferred; no lubricant if dry hands.	Patient undressed and in bed. Bench on which patient lies 60 cm. high, approachable from all sides. Masseur sits or stands beside it. Lower part of arm — patient and physical therapist sit on opposite sides of bench, patient's arm	Important; no hard and fast rule. Local—15 minutes; general—½ hour.	Daily; in acute injuries, sometimes several times daily.

Kleen — continued:		Friction—quite hard pressure.		Also use instruments and apparatus for vibration.	resting on bench. Throat or neck— patient sits on bench; physical therapist stands at front, side, or back.		
Lucas-Championnière (1843-1913)	Usually centrifugal (no deviation in direction, once established).	"Little more than a caress."	Slow and uniform. Rhythmical repetition.				
Hoffa (1859-1907)	Friction — circular. Pétrissage — from insertion to origin of muscle. Two-hand transverse to muscle fiber.	Friction — seeks to penetrate deeply. Pétrissage — hand presses firmly against belly of muscle. Correct amount can be judged only by practice. Grasp must be gentle, sympathetic, yet of sufficient firmness. New patients and painful cases, begin with little force and increase gradually.		Powder preferred.	Entire length of part supported so that muscles are relaxed. Patient sits on stool for massage of hand, neck, shoulder, and upper arm. For elbow, forearm, hand, and fingers, parts should rest on a table. For leg and foot, masseur sits opposite the patient, foot supported in his lap. Patient lies down for back, abdomen, thighs, or knee joints; thigh, masseur sits beside patient. Details of change in position of patient and masseur for various muscle groups of the thigh are given. Illustrations in 1897 edition show both patient and masseur seated for massage of elbow, shoulders, and neck; for foot, knee and thigh, patient is seated on table and masseur seated with patient's foot in his lap. Height of table should be somewhat above the knee of the operator and his position should be comfortable and not strained.	Local — 10-20 minutes. General — 30-45 minutes.	Daily

TABLE VII. *Components of Massage Techniques—Continued*

Name	Direction	Pressure	Rate and Rhythm	Medium	Position of Patient and Physical Therapist	Duration	Frequency
Kellogg (1852-1943)	Stroking, friction, and pétrissage — centripetal.	Friction — considerable pressure on thick masses, light on bony and thin tissues. Percussion — varying degrees of force. Deep kneading varies with tissues. Fist kneading — greatest degree force and pressure communicated to deepest part. Rolling and wringing sufficient to keep hand from slipping on skin. Tolerance of pressure established by prolonged treatment, gentle at beginning of treatment, gradually increased until almost the whole strength might be employed without injuring the patient.	Depends on type of movement. Stroking — not more than 1 or 2 inches per second. Friction — 30-180 strokes per minute, varying with length of stroke. Pétrissage — not too rapid, 30-90 per minute, more rapid in small parts. Wringing — not to exceed 30 per minute.	For reflex stroking — fingernail, end of lead pencil, wooden toothpick, or head of pin.			
Zabludowski (1851-1906)	Centripetal (return with light stroke).	Most cases should not be painful. When necessarily painful, pain should subside shortly. Criticism of Championnière's gentleness in massage: "Massage which	Determined by area covered. Beginning usually measured, swelling to speed, ending more slowly. Rhythm important, may be cultivated by practice with metronome.	Lard, powder, soapsuds, lanolin oil, creams, white Virginia petrolatum preferred.	Relaxation of all the body important. Position of patient depends on parts treated. Some work can be done in the standing position. Small children can be held in the lap if no table is avail-	5-30 minutes, varying with size of area, age of patient, duration of illness, constitution and	Usually daily, depending on physical and phychological reactions. Entire period usually 2-3 weeks.

Zabludowski — continued.	becomes painless ceases to be massage, only treatment by suggestion.			able. Support given by sound side; by hand of masseur while massaging with the other. Masseur should stand at back or side of patient for most work. He should have a sure footing. Posture is important for his own and the patient's confidence. This is best in the standing position. If he is sitting, the elbow (when arms flexed) should be above the area treated. Co-ordinated movement recommended for the masseur to avoid flexing and extending many joints.		
Mitchell (1859–1917)	Light if patient is apprehensive.	Slow if patient is apprehensive. Effleurage — return stroke faster than upward.	None, except in special circumstances (promotes growth of hair). If any used, suggests wool fat or oil of sweet almonds, but only on dry scaly skin or on the emaciated and elderly.	Patient reclines; physical therapist stands at patient's side or foot of bed. In some positions, physical therapist sits on table.	Depends on condition of patient. Local — 5-15 minutes; general — 50-60 minutes.	2-4 times daily.

TABLE VII. *Components of Massage Techniques—Continued*

Name	Direction	Pressure	Rate and Rhythm	Medium	Position of Patient and Physical Therapist	Duration	Frequency
Despard (published 1910)	Friction — circular. Effleurage — centripetal. Pétrissage — centripetal. Soothing stroking — centrifugal. Colon — along course.	Soothing stroking — gentle. Stimulating effect — strong. Vigor regulated by condition of patient.	Soothing stroking — slow. Stimulating stroking — quick. Rhythm important in all movements.	Dry rubbing preferred. Lubricant for young children, rickety subjects, old and emaciated persons, stiff joints, limbs previously in splints, skin dry, sensitive, or hairy. Suggested lubricants: coconut butter, olive oil, Neat's foot oil, white petrolatum, lanolin; dry hands; powder: talc or boric acid.	Patient in comfortable position. For back stroking, either prone, sitting, or standing with hands resting against the wall or other support. Masseur's position convenient for carrying out many manipulations. Should support the limbs except in percussion. General massage— describes position of patient for each area and position of masseur in relation to the patient when treating each area.	Definite periods, varying for each area and increasing under improvement. Varies 5-20 minutes.	
Bucholz (1874-)	Effleurage — with lymphatic flow (return lightly). Pétrissage — each manipulation centripetal. Succession of manipulations may be centripetal or centrifugal.	Effleurage at distal part of muscle, slight; increase over fleshy part; decrease at proximal. Moderate, fine, delicate touch more important than athletic hand.	Shaking — quick. Vibration — quick. Irritable cases — slow. Kneading depends on desired effects. Healthy persons 50-60 times per minute. Important in pétrissage. Shaking, and vibration quick rhythm.	Use common sense. For mild effleurage or large areas of dry skin — cold cream, petrolatum. Kneading and friction — no medium.	Patient in comfortable position, one which will allow operator to work with sufficient comfort. Muscles of patient should be relaxed, his joints held in middle position. Patient may be either in sitting or lying position for treating arms and shoulders, but for the rest of the body he should be lying. Does not favor sitting position for treating the legs, although it may be used for the foot and calf if the patient is sitting on a table and the operator in front of him on a chair.	Dependent on desired effect. Increase dependent on patient's reaction. Fresh injury — 5-10 minutes; general — 40-50 minutes.	Dependent on patient's social condition. Surgical cases twice daily.

| Mennell (1880-1957) | Friction – circular, superficial stroking direction of minor importance, but once established must be continued. Deep stroking – centripetal. Kneading – begin proximal; deep pressure, centripetal. | Amount dependent solely on relaxation of musculature; when relaxed, slight pressure will reach even deeper than when not. Kneading – greatest pressure when hand is at lowest part of circle, least when at opposite. Superficial stroking – gentle, sufficient only to ensure the patient's consciousness of the passage of the hand throughout the movement. Frictions – initially light, slowly and progressively increased. Gentleness essential to success. | Excessive rapidity inimical to success. Superficial stroking – slow, 15 times per minute (shoulder to hand). Slowness indispensable to rhythm and gentleness. Deep stroking – slow, to coordinate with normal flow of venous blood and lymph. Kneading – rapidity inimical to success. Friction – slow, unbroken rhythm essential. No time lag between end of stroke and commencement of next. Frictions – slow and unbroken. | Personal factor. French chalk and oil, soap and water. Oil on hard scaly skin. | Dependent entirely on results attained. Neurasthenia – initial 20 minutes; increase to 75 minutes; gradually decrease in similar manner. |

chapter 3

principles
of massage

The value of any treatment depends on a knowledge of its indications, the effects which will be produced by prescribing treatment, an understanding of the principles of the treatment, and the method of its application. Massage, like any other form of treatment, is not beneficial in all diseases or all injuries under all circumstances.

INDICATIONS FOR MASSAGE

The indications for the use of massage can be appreciated only by one who knows the anatomy and physiology of the human body and the processes of disease and injury. Only the physician who has made a diagnosis can determine whether or not massage will be an aid in his treatment of the patient. To make this decision, he must have a knowledge of the effects of massage and an understanding of the principles and methods of its application.

The therapeutic value of massage has often not been recognized because inadequately trained persons were not able to give adequate massage treatment with technique based on scientific knowledge. Since few physicians can devote the time necessary for the actual application of massage, they depend upon the physical therapist who is trained in its principles and technique to make the application of the treatment.

When administered intelligently and scientifically, with a thorough understanding of its limitations and of the dangers to be expected from its improper use, as well as the benefits derived when correctly applied, massage now plays an important part in medical treatment.

To obtain satisfactory results from the use of massage, it is necessary to realize that it is not a panacea and that it must be used correctly and used only in the treatment of the diseases and types of injuries in which benefit can reasonably be expected. Massage definitely may be either beneficial or harmful; it may be either indicated or contraindicated in the treatment of any condition. Mennell* stated, "Massage is a potent therapeutic agency, but misapplied it can result in a very serious evil." Failure to recognize this fact has been a cause of the misuse of massage in many instances and has resulted in the lack of appreciation of its value and in the neglect of its use in conditions for which it can be greatly beneficial.

Mennell stated, "Never yet was function restored by massage. In many cases, by its means, recovery will be hastened; in a few cases it may render recovery possible; but very rarely, if ever, will it suffice to cure" and "We must consider it entirely as a means to an end, that end being restoration of function." Massage is a valuable part of the treatment of the patient in many types of conditions both medical and surgical; however, it is only one of the physical therapy procedures which may be used. The relationship of massage to other forms of physical therapy as well as to the total treatment of the patient must be understood in order to avoid its misuse.

---

*Mennell, J. B.: Physical Treatment. 5th Ed. London, J. & A. Churchill Ltd., 1945.

PRESCRIPTION FOR MASSAGE

The physician is qualified to diagnose and to prescribe treatment. As he knows the indications for massage, only he should prescribe it. No therapist should administer a massage treatment without a definite prescription from a physician.

Mennell stated, "When a medical man orders massage, he should not try to hand over his responsibility to the masseur. He should consider the prescription of massage treatment in the same light as he would consider that of a potent drug and watch its effects no less closely, varying the dose and the nature of the dose from time to time according to indications.... But if he is to prescribe and intelligently watch his prescription, it is essential that he should render his instructions intelligible to his masseur, should know what effect he hopes to see and of what danger signals he must be aware."

In referring to prescription of massage, Jessie Wright stated, "Physical therapy should be prescribed with the same thought and precision as when selecting and dosing drugs.... In ordering massage, definite designation should be given as to the effect desired, exact areas to be covered, and whether superficial or deep movements are indicated.... As long as the therapist understands the purpose and effect desired, the choice of maneuvers and the details of the treatment usually may be left to her judgment, provided she has had approved training and experience."[80]

Elkins agreed with these authorities in stating, "In order for a physician adequately to prescribe massage, he should be aware of the types of massage used for therapeutic purposes, the proper methods of administering it, and be able to recognize good technic.[75]

Unfortunately, at the present time such ideal prescription of massage is not given by all those physicians who appreciate its beneficial effects and who prescribe it for the treatment of their patients. This places greater responsibility upon the therapist. If adequate and detailed prescription for massage has not been given, it is the responsibility of the therapist to consult with the physician and to ascertain his wishes in regard to the treatment. Information regarding the diagnosis and the effects desired from the treatment are essential. Mennell stated, "The prescription of details of techniques and of treatment should not be necessary, and, unless possessed of unusual knowledge and experience, most medical men will be wise if they leave these to the masseur. But, in order to decide upon the details, the masseur must know the nature of the conditions he is called upon to treat, and this means he must be provided with an accurate diagnosis."

It is absolutely necessary that there be close cooperation between the therapist who is applying the treatment and the physician who is responsible for the care of the patient and is prescribing the treatment. The therapist, because of the usually longer and more frequent contact with the patient, can be of valuable assistance to the physician by intelligently observing the patient's reaction to the treatment and reporting this to him. The therapist must necessarily have adequate knowledge of the tissues under treatment, of the pathology which exists, of the effects of massage, and of the technique of massage so that he can intelligently apply the treatment and make a report of his observations.

The therapist should at no time change an order which has been given for massage. He should, however, report to the physician if, from his observation of the patient's reactions, he believes that the physician might wish to change the prescription. Such reports may also be helpful to the physician by providing pertinent information which may affect his total treatment plan for the patient. The therapist may offer suggestions, provided he is ready to explain the reasons upon which they are based.

DOSAGE

Although many factors enter into the determination of the dosage for each individual patient, the prime factors are the pathology which exists and the results which are expected from the application of the massage. The components of technique which regulate the dosage of massage are: (1) duration, (2) frequency, and (3) type of movement.

While the dosage for a massage treatment should be prescribed by a physician, because of the many variable factors which regulate dosage it seems impossible to include all details of the treatment in the prescription. The physician is rarely if ever in constant attendance during the entire massage treatment; therefore, many of the details of the treatment must be left to the judgment of the therapist. Such judgment can be developed only with adequate fundamental knowledge of anatomy, physiology, and pathology together with a thorough understanding of the basic principles of massage. In addition, it is necessary that the techniques of massage be applied thoughtfully and intelligently.

Duration

The duration of any massage treatment will depend upon: (a) the area to be treated, (b) the rate of the movements, (c) the age and size of the individual, and (d) changes in symptoms.

AREA

The duration of the treatment obviously will vary according to the size of the area to be treated. This area should be indicated in the prescription. Although the actual pathology which exists may be localized to a small area, there undoubtedly will be disturbances of physiology in the adjacent region. Therefore, the treatment should not be limited to the diseased or injured area only.

Unfortunately, the therapist is not always given enough information in the prescription. For example, a prescription may be given for massage for pain in, or injury to, "the shoulder." The intelligent physical therapist will know that this does not imply that only the shoulder joint is to be included in the treatment but that also, in order to make the treatment effective, at least all of the muscles controlling the movement at the shoulder joint should be included. In addition, the circulation of the arm, forearm, and hand may be impaired, and spasm and edema may be present. Under such conditions, the physical therapist should consult the physician for more specific instructions.

It is the custom in some prescriptions to establish an approximate length of time for a treatment. The time which frequently is given for an upper extremity is from ten to fifteen minutes, for a lower extremity, fifteen to twenty minutes, and from fifteen to twenty minutes for a back. The approximate time usually allowed for massage to the entire body is from forty-five minutes to one hour. If such practice is rigidly adhered to, it would seen impossible to accomplish the best results.

RATE OF MOVEMENTS

The rate of the movements will effect the total amount of massage applied within a given time. A definite uniform rate should be established for all movements so that the dosage may be evaluated.

Mennell stressed that massage movements (except percussion) should be slow, gentle, and rhythmical. He gave a rate of about 15 strokes a minute for stroking from hand to shoulder. Beard and Wood determined that when the hand or hands move over the tissues at approximately *seven inches per second* the desired effects, both mechanical and reflex, can be obtained. This rate, which is the equivalent of Mennell's rate as stated above, should be applied not only to stroking movements but also the gliding and circular movements of kneading and the circular movements of friction.

SIZE AND AGE OF PATIENT

The size and age of the patient will also affect the duration of the treatment. With a constant rate of massage, a shorter length of time will be necessary to treat a comparatively small person because the amount of tissues being manipulated is less than for a large person.

Mennell belived that the duration of massage for the very young or the aged should be curtailed, as the reflex arc is more sensitive and the fullest effect is secured rapidly; this is particularly true if the aim of the massage is entirely to secure a reflex effect. For these individuals, one should reduce the number of movements rather than increase the rate of movements (a practice which is sometimes thoughtlessly followed, and which defeats the purpose of the massage).

Various medical authorities, in discussing dosage of massage, recognize the variability of application and the difficulty in prescribing specific doses. It would seem impossible to avoid either insufficient treatment or overdose if a certain, specified length of time is allotted for each treatment.

Mennell emphasized the importance of intelligent observation of the patient by the therapist during treatment and the danger of an overdose in treatment as well as the futility of an underdose. He believed, however, that unless at some time there is evidence of an overdose, it may be quite possible that an insufficient amount of treatment has been given. This emphasizes the necessity of constant and intelligent observation of the patient and his reaction to the treatment.

CHANGES IN SYMPTOMS

As the condition of the treated tissue changes, it may be necessary to make a change in the duration of the treatment. Keeping in mind that massage is "a means to an end," the duration of the massage may be gradually shortened as the treatment is successful in accomplishing the desired results. If the massage has not accomplished the desired results, it may be that the duration has not been sufficiently long or that an overdose has been given. The therapist should closely observe the patient to appreciate the need for the change, and adapt the duration of treatment to the need. If the physician is not in constant or frequent observation of the patient during treatment, the therapist should report to him the patient's reaction to the treatment and also his progress, or lack of it.

The duration of any massage treatment, therefore, should vary according to the pathology which is present and the size of the area to be treated, the rate of speed of the movements, the age of the patient, and any change in symptoms. To obtain the maximum benefit from any massage treatment and to avoid inadequate treatment or an overdose in duration, it is essential that the physical therapist have good scientific knowledge of massage and of its physiological effects and that he thoughtfully and intelligently apply the massage, observing carefully the effects of the treatment.

Frequency

The frequency of massage should definitely be included in the prescription. The frequency of application, as in all factors of dosage, will depend upon the pathological condition which is to be treated. It is generally believed that massage is most effective when administered daily, although some investigators have suggested that it is more beneficial when administered more frequently and for a shorter duration than would be advisable for a once-daily treatment. Daily administration is customary, especially when the treatment is first instituted, and as the patient's condition improves the dosage may be decreased by less frequent application.

Although the ideal treatment for every patient is the aim of all medical personnel, unfortunately it is not always possible. Massage treatment is a time-consuming, and therefore an expensive, form of treatment and the economic status of the patient must at times be given consideration. If necessary, it may be advisable to administer the treatment at less frequent intervals. The physician will be familiar with the circumstances and will prescribe the frequency of treatment which he believes is most beneficial for each patient.

Type of Movement

In relation to dosage, there is little if any scientific information regarding differences in the effect of the various types of massage movements. Until such information is obtained by scientific research, it is necessary, therefore, in this as well as in many other forms of medical treatment, to rely upon clinical evidence. If there is a difference in the effect of the various types of movements, it is evident that the selection of the movement used should be based on its effect upon the pathology which exists and the results which are desired.

Therefore, it will be necessary to regulate the dosage by the selection of the type of movement which will be most effective. For example, a type of movement such as deep stroking, which may effectively increase the venous and lymphatic flow, may not be as effective in the treatment of an indurated area as a deep kneading movement. The therapist should be able to give in detail the reasons for each massage movement used during a treatment—why one movement is given in preference to another in that particular instance, the duration of each type of movement, what effect is anticipated, and how that effect is to be attained.

The dosage may be varied by the manner in which the different types of movements are applied. It is difficult to evaluate accurately the amount of pressure which is used, but the effect obtained will depend to a great extent upon the regulation of the pressure and the stimulation which it produces. Deep pressure may produce a strong stimulation and an increase in tension and pain, while lighter pressure may produce a mild stimulation, relaxation, and diminished pain. The reaction to external stimulation will vary with different individuals and with the pathology of the tissues under treatment. The duration and frequency of treatment and the type of movement selected will depend in general upon the pathology which exists and the effect expected from the treatment.

Thoughtful observation of the reaction of the patient and of the local effects produced must be constant, and the type of movement and the pressure regulated accordingly. Unless massage is thoughtfully and intelligently applied, its use becomes empirical.

If the therapist is absorbed in irrelevant matters such as conversation with a patient, such concentration on the treatment is impossible and may lead to a useless or even harmful performance of movements without accomplishing the desired results.

CLASSIFICATION AND DESCRIPTION OF MASSAGE MOVEMENTS

Mennell classified all massage movements under three simple headings: stroking, compression, and percussion.

In order to avoid confusion and to clarify terminology, this general classification will be used. All movements may be varied by pressure, direction, and the part of the hand used in application. A uniform rate of speed should be established for all massage, and an even rhythm maintained throughout the movement.

Stroking

A stroking movement consists of the passage of the hand, or parts therof, over a comparatively extended area of the body; the pressure maintained is more or less constant throughout the stroke. Any degree of pressure may be applied, varying from the lightest possible touch to very deep pressure.

SUPERFICIAL STROKING

A superficial stroke is performed with extremely light pressure, using the entire palmar surface of the hand. The fingers are held together, and the thumb is abducted (Fig. 1) or adducted (Fig. 2) as necessary to increase or lessen the area of palmar surface to fit the part of the body which is being massaged. One or both hands may be used (Figs. 1, 2, 3).

Mennel learned from Lucas-Championnière the value of very light stroking movements, "little more than a caress." This form of massage is simple, yet it is difficult to perform. It requires a certain skillful technique of application in order to obtain

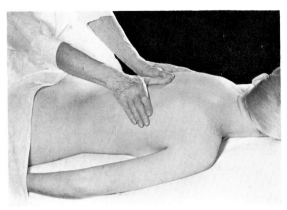

Figure 1

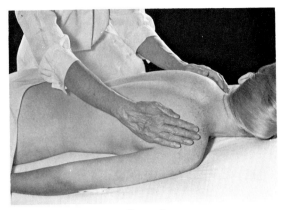

Figure 2

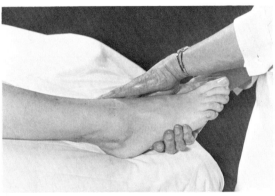

Figure 3

the desired soothing reflex effect. Relaxation of contracted muscles may be obtained and muscle spasm overcome through the reflex response to superficial stroking when correct technique has been employed. The attainment of this technique requires long practice with careful attention to the following four points:

Pressure

The pressure must be very light. Making and breaking contact of the hand with the skin at the beginning and end of the movement must be so gentle and gradual that it is almost imperceptible to the patient. The hand must be flexible and under perfect control so that its entire palmar surface will be in contact and conform to the contour of the area being massaged, so that the pressure is equal at all points.

Direction

The movement may be given in any desired direction, as the pressure is so light that it does not directly affect the circulation. In fact, the wishes of the patient may be followed as to what is most restful and soothing to him. For the limbs, the stroke is usually in the centrifugal direction. The growth of hair naturally falls in this direction, and stroking performed in an opposite direction is unpleasant. The direction of the movement, once established, should be continued throughout the treatment.

In certain instances, especially when the patient is apprehensive, and sensitive areas are to be massaged, it may be of advantage to change from superficial stroking to deep stroking by gradually increasing the pressure. In such a case the superficial stroking should be given in the centripetal direction.

Rhythm

Even rhythm is essential to secure relaxation. It is established by making the time for each stroke and the time between successive strokes the same. Good rhythm can be attained only by the physical therapist's assuming a comfortable position of his entire body, thus allowing well controlled movements of his arms and hands. Repeated practice is required. It may be of assistance, when learning, to count in rhythm and time the movements to the count.

Rate of Movement

The established rate (see p. 38) must be constant throughout the stroke, while the hand is in contact with the skin and while it is in the air for the return movement. This rate should be practiced by the physical therapist until it is instinctively carried out through all massage.

DEEP STROKING

Any stroking movement which is given with sufficient pressure to produce mechanical as well as reflex effects is classified as deep stroking, even though the pressure may be very slight. The purpose of deep stroking massage is to assist the venous and lymphatic circulation by its mechanical effects on the tissues.

Deep stroking may be performed with any part of one hand or with both hands, depending upon the area being massaged. Usually one uses the palmar surface of the whole hand, fingers, or thumb. The part of the hand used is kept in contact at the end of the stroke and returned over the same area with a superficial stroke. The purpose of keeping the hand in contact for the return stroke is to avoid the reflex stimulus to the nerve endings in the skin caused by breaking and again making contact with the skin. There is no particular benefit from the return stroke itself, but if the pressure is as light as that of a superficial stroke it does not interfere with the mechanical effect of the deep stroke upon the flow of blood and lymph. Some authorities do not agree that the hand should remain in contact during the return stroke, but in the author's experience it has been found to be less irritating to the patient than the frequent make and break of contact.

In order to apply this type of massage effectively, it is essential to have the patient's muscles relaxed; to consider the effect of gravity; to regulate pressure according to the bulk and condition of the muscle; and to make the pressure in the general direction of venous and lymphatic flow. It is important to have all the muscles of the area to be treated, and those proximal to it, relaxed, as a contracted muscle will lessen the lumen of the veins and defeat the chief purpose of this type of massage. Superficial stroking may be used as a preliminary to deep stroking to gain relaxation of the muscles. To obtain complete relaxation, the patient must be in a comfortable recumbent position. Also with the patient recumbent, the effect of gravity in the venous and lymphatic circulations is decreased.

The technique of deep stroking requires careful attention to the following four points:

Pressure

The use of the term deep stroking does not necessarily imply that force should be used; the pressure required may be very slight. The term is used in contrast to superficial stroking, which has only a reflex effect. The hands must be flexible and conform to the contour of the area under treatment so that the pressure is transmitted to all the structures under the hand. The pressure must be even throughout the movement. The physical therapist must keep in mind that the tissues he is massaging are structures which can easily be irritated or injured. Heavy, forceful pressure is not only unnecessary but may even be harmful. The efficacy of the stroking may be reduced by reflex protective muscle spasm as the result of pain, and tissues can be bruised by uneven pressure or by too heavy pressure upon small areas.

Direction

For the reasons stated (see pages 49, 50, 51) the direction of deep stroking of the limbs should be centripetal. The hand is kept in contact after the deep stroke is finished and returned with a superficial stroke to the distal portion of the area being treated. The deep stroke is then repeated without any interruption of contact or change in the rate of movement.

Rhythm

An even rhythm must be maintained throughout the movement of deep stroking for the same reasons as given under superficial stroking. While the objective in deep stroking is primarily for a mechanical effect, the reflex effect of contact of the hand cannot be disregarded. If the rhythm is uneven, it may cause a protective reflex response.

Rate of Movement

The established rate of movement (see page 38) should be maintained for deep stroking. There is no advantage in rapidity of movement, as the flow of blood in the veins and of the lymph in its channels is comparatively slow. Only by using a slow rate of movement can the purpose of this form of massage be accomplished.

Compression

A compression movement consists of repeatedly grasping and releasing the tissues with one or both hands or parts thereof, in a lifting, rolling, or pressing movement. The outstanding characteristic of this movement, as contrasted to stroking movements, is that the pressure is applied intermittently.

The purposes of compression movements are to stretch shortened tissues, to loosen adherent tissues, and to hasten the venous and lymphatic flow.

Compression movements are classified as (a) kneading and (b) friction.

KNEADING

A kneading movement consists of grasping or compressing a muscle group, a muscle, or part of a muscle and applying pressure, then releasing the pressure, progressing to an adjacent area, and repeating the process. This movement may be performed with one (Fig. 4) or both hands (Fig. 5) using the palm, the palmar surface

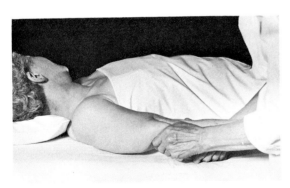

Figure 4

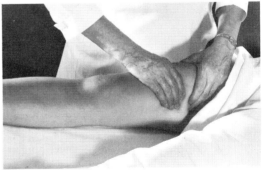

Figure 5

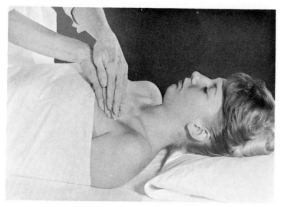

Figure 6

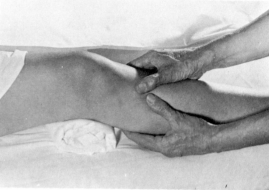

Figure 7

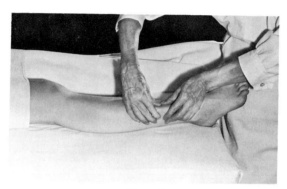

Figure 8

of the fingers (Fig. 6), the thumb (Fig. 7), or thumb and fingers (Fig. 8). Kneading movements are classified according to the part of the hand used (for example, palmar kneading and thumb kneading).

The essential requirements for effective kneading are: to have the patient in a comfortable, relaxed position; to make use of the assistance of gravity; to perform the movements slowly, gently and rhythmically; and to make the part of the hand that is used conform to the contour of the area. Relaxation of the muscles is important for the reasons given under *deep stroking* (see pages 42 and 49–51).

Some authorities believe this form of massage is more effective in aiding absorption of substances within the tissues than is deep stroking. In the author's experience this has often been clinically demonstrated.

The following points must be considered when kneading movements are used:

Pressure

Although the pressure is intermittent, great care must be used in this movement to avoid pinching the skin and superficial tissues. To avoid this, the pressure should be gradually reduced as the bulk of the tissues diminishes.

If the muscles are relaxed, the pressure should not be extremely heavy for the reasons given on pages 49–51.

Direction

The direction of these movements is significant only as it is related to the purpose for which the massage is being given. For example, in treating an extremity the massage may be started at the proximal part and each succeeding movement performed over the more immediate distal area. In this instance the hand (or part thereof which is used) returns to the proximal part with a deep stroke. In another instance, the movement may be started at the distal part of the extremity and each succeeding movement performed over the immediate, more proximal area. This time the hand (or part thereof) returns to the distal part with a superficial stroke. *In either case the direction of the heavy pressure of each individual kneading movement must always be in the centripetal direction.*

Rhythm and Rate of Movement

The same even rhythm and rate of movement should be observed in all kneading movements as has been established in stroking movements.

FRICTION

The purpose of friction movements are to loosen adherent skin, loosen scars, free adhesions of deeper structures, and aid in the absorption of local effusion around the joints.

Friction may be performed with the whole or the proximal part of the palm of the hand (Fig. 9), or with the palmar surface of the distal phalanx of the thumb (Figs. 10 and 11), or of the fingers (Fig. 12).

The superficial tissues are moved over the underlying structures by keeping the hand or part thereof in firm contact with the skin and making circular movements over

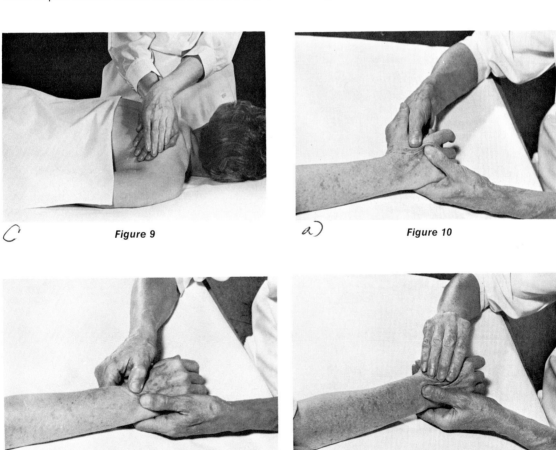

Figure 9

Figure 10

Figure 11

Figure 12

a limited area. Only after several circles over this area have been completed is the pressure released so that the hand can (without losing contact) glide to the next area and repeat the movement.

Pressure

The pressure applied in friction movements should be firm but not so heavy as to cause injury to the underlying structures.

Direction

Although the movement is in a circular direction, the pressure of the movement must be applied in the direction which will produce tension on the involved structures and thereby stretch and loosen them.

Rhythm and Rate of Movement

The same even rhythm and rate of movement should be observed in friction as in other movements.

To perform friction, either one or both hands may be used. For example:
  (a) Two thumbs may work closely together, alternating the movements (Fig. 10).
  (b) One thumb may give support and the other thumb work against it as it does the friction movement (Fig. 11).
  (c) Over a large, flat surface, one palm does the friction movement, reinforced by the other hand (Fig. 9).
  (d) The fingers of one hand may work against the support of the thumb, while the other hand supports or stabilizes the part of the body (Fig. 12).

Percussion and Vibration

Percussive movements are a series of brief, brisk, rapidly applied contacts of the hand, or hands in alternating movements. They are classified as hacking (with the ulnar border of the hand), clapping or cupping (using fingers, thumb and palm together to form a concave surface—see Fig. 13), tapping (with the tips of the fingers), and beating (fists half closed).

Clapping (cupping) is a technique of major importance when used in the treatment of patients with respiratory problems. (See p. 147).

Percussive movements other than clapping (cupping) are usually used on healthy individuals and have little place in the treatment of pathological conditions. They have been recommended for obtaining reflex muscle contraction and increased capillary

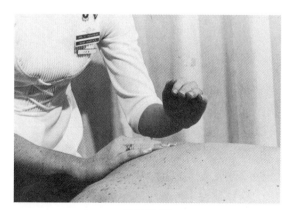

Figure 13

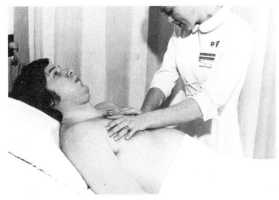

Figure 14A

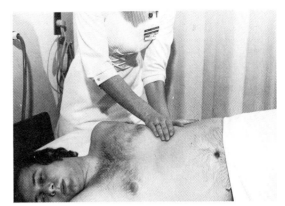

Figure 14B

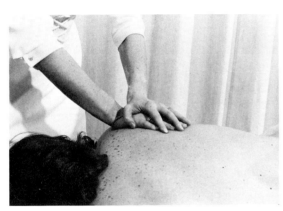

Figure 15

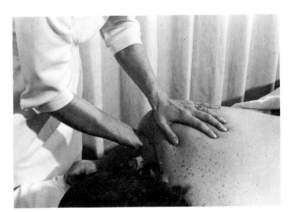

Figure 16

circulation, but there are other more efficient and more effective physical therapy measures for obtaining these results.

Shaking and vibration are techniques for gross and more refined vibratory effects on tissues. In both types of movements the hands remain in contact with the tissues, and the shaking or fine vibration is initiated in the therapist's own movements and transmitted to the patient via the therapist's hands, which are already in contact with the skin. Shaking is used therapeutically on patients with mobile chest walls (see Fig. 14), and vibration (see Figs. 15 and 16) is often a vital component in the treatment of respiratory conditions, by itself and in conjunction with clapping (cupping) and other measures (see pp. 146, 147). In contrast to the percussive movements, the techniques of applying vibration skillfully requires strenuous muscular effort on the part of the therapist, with precise control of this effort as its force is transmitted to the patient.

chapter 4

effects of massage

Massage produces mechanical stimulation to the tissues by means of rhythmically applied pressure and stretching. Pressure compresses soft tissues and distorts the nerve-ending networks of receptors; stretching applies tension on soft tissues and also distorts the nerve-ending plexuses of receptors. Use of these two forces can, by changing the lumen of blood vessels and lymph vessel spaces, affect capillary, venous, arterial, and lymphatic circulation. We can demonstrate axon reflex. We can stimulate exteroceptors, both superficial and deep, in the skin; proprioceptors in the muscles and tendons; and interoceptors in the deeper tissues of the body. We can loosen mucus and promote drainage of excess fluids from the lungs.

How these mechanical forces are applied is determined by the therapist in his choice of massage movements (stroking friction, kneading, percussion and vibration) and his skill in regulating the duration, quality, intensity, and rhythm of the stimulus (see Chapter 3, page 37). What effects massage may have are not as well understood or as well defined. Many claims have been made for the use of massage (see Chapter 2). Some are based upon clinical experience, both objective reports and "testimonials." Some are rationalizations of hypotheses based on knowledge of anatomy and physiology. Some are based on controlled, carefully worked out laboratory studies, and some on what might be described as "wishful thinking." Comparatively little has been written, and relatively few studies have been made, on massage.

In a review of the literature of the last ten years (1963–72) we found that studies were done by Severini and Venerando[67, 68] on effects of massage on the cardiovascular system in 1967; Bell[4] reported in 1964 on the results of a study on changes in blood volume following massage; Barr and Taslitz[2] (1967) did a well controlled study on the effects of back massage on the autonomic system; Bork, Karling and Faust[9] reported in 1971 on the effects of whole body massage on serum enzyme levels.

CLASSIFICATIONS OF MASSAGE EFFECTS

Effects of massage have been described and classified in several different ways. Mennell referred to mechanical (pressure and tension), chemical, reflex, and psychological effects. Other authors discussed general and local effects. These effects might also be classified as physical, physiological (including reflex), and psychological.

A purely physical effect can be demonstrated by stroking superficial veins and, with direct pressure, removing the blood from the portion of the vein which is stroked.

Lucas-Championnière's technique of obtaining relaxation of muscles in spasm following a fracture by superficial stroking can be explained only as a reflex (physiological) effect.[54]

Mennell's caution about "rubbing a disability into a patient's mind," when massaging a part which has sustained a minor injury, stresses a purely psychological effect.

It is probable, however, that most massage treatments produce their effects as the result of a combination of physical, physiological, and psychological factors.

Effects on Circulation of Blood

Mennell believed that it is impossible to assist the arterial circulation directly by mechanical effects of massage.

He theorized that pressure by massage in the direction of the venous flow is comparable to squeezing any soft tube to empty it of fluid. If the muscles are relaxed, they constitute a soft mass containing tubes which are filled with fluid. Any pressure applied to the mass should push the fluid in these tubes in the direction which the pressure is applied; therefore, the deeper veins will also be emptied if sufficient pressure is applied to the entire mass. Such pressure might at the same time retard the rate of arterial blood flow if it is heavy enough to compress the arteries as well as the veins.

Theoretically, if the amount of venous blood brought to the heart can be increased by massage, the rate of the heart beat or the stroke volume might be increased and thus a greater amount of arterial blood be carried to the periphery. However, there is little evidence of such a simple mechanical reaction of the arterial and arteriolar system to massage. Wakim and co-workers found that there was "no consistent or significant average increase in total blood flow" in normal, rheumatoid arthritic, or spastic persons following deep stroking and kneading massage. There was "moderate, consistent, and definite increase in circulation" after such massage to flaccid paralyzed extremities. "Vigorous, stimulating massage resulted in consistent and significant increases in average blood flow of the massaged extremity" but produced no change in blood flow in the contralateral unmassaged extremity.

According to Pemberton,[63] the nervous system, probably through the sympathetic division, contributes to a reflex influence on the blood vessels of the parts concerned. He believed that it is probable, therefore, that vessels within the muscular system or elsewhere are emptied during massage not alone by virtue of being squeezed but also through this reflex action.

Pemberton stated that microscopic observation of fields in which only a few capillaries are open, and hence in which only a few can be seen, reveals that massage may cause almost all the smaller vessels to become visible because of the blood flow created through them.

Although there is little information on the type of massage that was used, several convincing experiments have been done which show that massage will increase the circulation of the blood.

Wolfson studied the effect of deep kneading massage on venous blood flow in normal dog limbs and found that massage caused a great initial increase with a fairly rapid decrease to a rate less than normal even before the end of stimulation. Immediately following the cessation of the procedure, he noted, the blood flow slowly increased again to normal rate. He concluded that the actual volume of blood, therefore, which passed through the limb during the period of stimulation and recovery is not greater than normal, but there is a more complete emptying for a short period of time, and therefore a greater supply of fresh blood is brought to the part. He suggested that it would seem logical to use short but frequent treatments of massage.

Carrier has shown that light pressure produces an almost instantaneous, though transient, dilatation of the capillary vessels, whereas heavier pressure may produce more enduring dilatation. Microscopic observation of fields in which only a few capillaries are open shows that pressure may cause nearly all the smaller vessels to become visible.

Pemberton[61] described the work of Clark and Swanson, who made cinematographic studies upon the capillary circulation in the ear of a rabbit, utilizing a permanent window for observation. These studies demonstrated that following massage more capillaries were opened with an increased rate of blood flow and a change in the blood vessel wall which was evidenced by the "sticking" and emigration of leucocytes.

That massage increases the blood flow also has been shown experimentally by Rosenthal[20] and by Brunton and Tunnicliffe.

It has been claimed that the reflex effect of superficial stroking will improve cutaneous circulation, especially the blood flow in superficial veins and lymphatics; aid in interchange of tissue fluids; increase nutrition of the tissues; and remove products of fatigue or inflammation. S. Wright stated in 1939 that these claims must be examined critically from the viewpoint of present-day knowledge of physiology.[63, 81] He maintained that it is difficult to make positive statements concerning reflex effects produced by massage with the few properly controlled clinical observations that are available and that the problem demanded further investigation.

Severini and Venerando[67] reported that superficial massage produced no significant changes other than in skin temperature. Deep massage caused an increase in blood flow, systolic stroke volume (hence in heart capacity) and oscillometric index, and a decrease in systolic and diastolic arterial pressure and pulse frequency. Deep massage led to an increase in blood flow and oscillometric index in the untreated homologous limb.

Bell's report stated that after deep stroking and kneading the calf of one leg for ten minutes, plethysmographic studies showed blood volume had doubled, thus doubling the rate of blood flow, an effect lasting 40 minutes, as contrasted with the effect of exercises when the rate of blood flow fell after 10 minutes.

The Barr and Taslitz[2] study showed that systolic and diastolic blood pressure tended to decrease after a 20 minute back massage, with a delayed effect of an increase in systolic pressure and a small additional decrease in diastolic pressure. The heart rate increased.

Severini and Venerando[68] combined massage with the use of a hyperemia-producing drug (containing vanellylon amide and butoxethyl nicotinate). The combined treatment led to a significant and prolonged rise of skin temperature. When the drug was used alone or with superficial massage there was no change in circulation in muscles, but with deep massage there was an appreciable and effective increase in blood flow in muscles.

Effects on Circulation of Lymph

In the lymphatic capillaries and plexuses of the skin and subcutaneous tissue, lymph can move in any direction. Its movement depends upon forces outside the lymphatic system. Its course is determined by such factors as gravity, muscle contraction, passive movement, or massage. If obstruction of the deeper lymphatics occurs in a part, it is still possible to keep the superficial lymphatics open and, if the part is massaged or given opportunity to drain by gravity, lymph will move through these other channels in the direction of the external force.

Animal experiments show that there is very little lymph flow when a muscle is at rest.[81] Cuthbertson describes von Mesengeil's and Kellgren and Colombo's studies on the effects of massage on the flow of lymph, which give evidence of the increase in lymph flow when the muscles have been massaged.

Von Mesengeil "repeatedly injected China ink into corresponding articulations of rabbits. One joint was massaged and the corresponding one left as a control. . . . In the legs without massage, the tendency of the colored material to pass toward the heart was very small, but in those legs subjected to massage there was great absorption of the ink above the joint in the intermuscular connective tissues and in the lymphatic glands. The lymphatics passing up to the glands were deeply stained black."

Kellgren and Colombo found that "massage always had a sure and effective influence in increasing the rapidity of the absorption of substances injected into animals in all the organs which can be subjected to manipulations—subcutaneous tissues, muscles, articulations, and serous cavities. . . . The course which the injected substance followed during its absorption was always that of the nearest lymphatics and the glands into which they pass. Deep effleurage (stroking) was probably less effective than the squeezing and rolling of muscles and subcutaneous tissue."

McMaster also found, by experiments in which the limbs of normal individuals were massaged after intradermal dye injections, that massage increased lymph flow.

Drinker and Yoffey cannulated the cervical lymph trunks in an anesthetized dog and were able to obtain a flow of lymph all day long by massaging the head and neck above the cannulae. When the massage was stopped, lymph flow either ceased or was negligible. They state that in treating chronic inflammatory conditions in which fibrosis is sure to advance if tissue fluid and lymph remain stagnant in the part, massage in the direction of lymph flow is preeminently the best artificial measure for moving extravascular fluid into lymphatics and for moving lymph onward toward the blood stream.

Drinker and Yoffey also found that the effects of posture were very obvious and that lymph flow from a dependent, quiescent part was practically negligible. Therefore, in order most efficiently to influence the flow of lymph in any area, it seemed logical that the part should be elevated during the application of massage.

Ladd, Kottke, and Blanchard compared the effects of massage, passive motion, and electrical stimulation on the rate of lymph flow in the forelegs of fifteen dogs and found that massage was "significantly more effective than either passive motion or electrical stimulation in this series of animals." All three procedures were found to increase the lymph flow greatly above that of the control period.

Bell recommended the use of massage for the treatment of edema of fractures because of its effect on venous and lymph flow.

Effects on Nervous System

Little information is available in the literature on the actual effects of massage upon the function of the nervous system.

Bucholz stated that it is impossible to show that massage produces any change in the nerve itself.

Chor and his associates[16] found that the degree of regeneration of a peripheral nerve which had been cut and sutured was not influenced by the use of massage and passive exercise.

Von Mesengeil[20] demonstrated clinically that the pain caused by vigorous massage was gradually lessened when the massage was continued for some time as compared to that caused at the beginning of the treatment. Although it frequently is possible, by massage, to relieve certain types of pain, no clear-cut explanation has been made as to how this is accomplished.

The sedative effect of a general massage can easily be demonstrated, and Mennell stated that "there is probably an effect on the central nervous system as well as a local effect on the sensory, and possibly the motor, nerves."

Experimental studies on reflex control of circulation[20, 52, 61] and neuromuscular responses[31, 65] give some support to hypotheses that massage has definite reflex effects[20, 25, 49, 54, 61] but many reflex effects seem to be hypothesized for want of any other rational explanation. Just what specific reflex mechanisms are responsible has not been made clear, nor how simple or complex the reflex action(s) may be. Much work needs to be done to clarify and verify these concepts by controlled clinical and laboratory studies, correlated with current physiological and neurophysiological concepts.

The work of Barr and Taslitz is an example of the kind of studies which can and need to be done for a variety of massage treatments. In addition to the effects of a 20 minute back massage on blood pressure and heart rate (see p. 50) Barr and Taslitz report an increase in skin sweating and thus a decreased resistance to galvanic current (galvanic skin response); after a slight decrease in body temperature (0° to 0.1°C) in the control period, an increase from 0° to 0.2°C at the end of the massage; and an increase in pupil diameter, which, in their opinion, may or may not have been a result of the massage. Their results indicate an increase in sympathetic activity in most indexes.

Effects on Muscle Tissue

The literature regarding the effects of massage contains a relatively large number of positive statements and implications regarding the effect of massage on the muscular system as compared to its effects on other systems and tissues of the body. Some of these statements cannot be substantiated by clinical observation or by scientific research.

NORMAL MUSCLES

Kellogg stated, "Massage produces an actual increase in the size of the muscle structures. The muscle is also found to become firmer and more elastic under its influence."

McMillan stated, "The muscles are strengthened and made to grow by manipulation."

According to Despard, "Massage improves the nutrition of the muscles and consequently promotes their development."

However, more recent authorities are generally agreed that massage will not increase muscle strength.

Although the theory that kneading a muscle ("working a muscle up") makes it stronger has been advanced, Mennell believed that this is a delusion which must be eradicated. He stated, "By one means alone can muscular strength be developed, and that is by muscular contraction, and no form of massage can do more than aid this means indirectly," and again. "To use massage aright we must consider it entirely as a means to an end, that end being restoration of function." As a means to an end, massage may be useful in making it possible for a muscle to perform more exercise and thereby develop its strength. This fact has been proven by experimental work done by Rosenthal, Mosso and Maggiora, and others.[20] They have shown that a muscle fatigued by work or by electrical stimulation will be restored much more rapidly and thoroughly by massage than by rest of the same duration.

Nordschow and Bierman did a study of twenty-five normal, healthy, active subjects to determine "whether manually applied massage could cause measurable muscle relaxation in the normal human subject." A "finger to floor" test was used to measure tension in the posterior muscles of the back, thighs, and legs, as each subject stood with knees straight and bent forward and touched or attempted to touch the floor with the finger tips. Following the attempt to touch the floor, each subject then assumed a comfortable, well-supported prone position for thirty minutes, and the "finger to floor" test was repeated. He then reassumed the prone position and was given thirty minutes of massage, fifteen to the back (similar to that described on pages 93–102 and 137–140), and seven and one half to the posterior aspects of each lower extremity (similar to that described on pages 125–126).

Three measurement scores were obtained for each individual. "Score 1: Distance in inches from the floor after rest minus the distance before rest. Score 2: The distance after massage, minus the distance after rest just before massage. Score 3: The distance after massage minus the distance before rest." The authors concluded that "manual massage can cause relaxation of voluntary muscles."

Bell reported that muscle fatigue was relieved more quickly by massage and rest than by rest alone, and suggests alternate "bouts" of exercise and massage in therapy (as is frequently done in sports).

The term "muscle tone" is used to describe the state in a muscle which gives it a quality of firmness. It has been defined as a state of constant contraction of a number of motor units in the muscles. Although some statements in literature imply that massage increases muscle tone, it has not been shown clinically or experimentally that this is true.

PATHOLOGICAL CONDITIONS IN MUSCLE

Experimental studies have been made of the effects of massage upon injured muscle and upon denervated muscle.

Injured Muscle

Castex[54] performed a series of experiments to show the effects of massage upon injured muscles. Animal muscles were subjected to crushing injury, massage was given to one group, and the other used as controls. The muscle tissue of both groups were later examined microscopically. Lucas-Championnière[54] summarized the results as follows:

"The untreated parts showed:

"i. Dissociation into fibrillae of the muscular fibers, as shown by well-marked longitudinal striation;

"ii. A hyperplasia, sometimes a simple thickening, of the connective tissue;

"iii. An increase in places of the number of nuclei in the connective tissue;

"iv. Interstitial hemorrhages;

"v. An enlargement of blood vessels, with hyperplasia of their adventitious coats;

"vi. The sarcolemma was usually intact, but, in one section, a multiplication of nuclei was seen, giving an appearance somewhat resembling an interstitial myositis."

"In the massaged limbs:

"i. The muscle appeared normal;

"ii. No secondary fibrous bands separated the muscle fibers;

"iii. There was no fibrous thickening around the vessels;

"iv. The general bulk of the muscles was greater;

"v. There were no signs of hemorrhages."

Denervated Muscle

Although massage has been used quite extensively in the treatment of denervated muscle, there is little information in literature concerning its effectiveness. Some studies have been made in an effort to determine its effect on the histopathological changes in the muscle itself, on atrophy, and on the strength of the muscle. However, the investigators have not agreed in their conclusions.

Chor et al.[16] conducted an experiment to study the effects of massage on atrophy and the histopathological changes which occur in denervated muscle.

Two groups of Macacus rhesus monkeys were subjected to unilateral section of the sciatic nerve, the nerves were immediately sutured, and the extremity was immobilized in a plaster cast. After a period of four weeks, massage (stroking and kneading) and passive motion were given for seven minutes daily to one group and the control group kept at complete rest. After a period of time varying from two months in some animals to six months in others, the muscles were examined microscopically to determine the histopathological changes. These were found to be similar to the changes found by Castex in injured muscles. The muscles kept at rest were pale and surrounded by thickened septums of fibrous tissue, with whitish and yellowish streaks throughout. Microscopically, this fibrosis was clearly demonstrable, both surrounding muscle fibers and replacing atrophied fibers.

The massaged muscles were supple and elastic, with considerably less fibrosis and adhesions.

The amount of restoration of muscle function after reinnervation is determined by the ratio of functioning muscle fibers to fibrous tissue which has replaced degenerated muscle fibers. Massage, by preventing to some extent the formation of inelastic fibrous tissue and adhesions, aided in maintaining a favorable ratio for greater recovery of function.

Chor and Doldkart[15] has previously studied atrophy of muscle from disuse and atrophy of denervated muscle. They observed that atrophy which occurs in a skeletal muscle not in use is slow and is associated with very simple structural changes. The loss of muscle bulk was accounted for on the basis of a diminished quantity of sarcoplasm in the individual muscle fibers. The atrophied muscle fibers are narrower and are packed more closely together. The characteristic cross striations persist. There is no actual degeneration of the muscle fibers. The intramuscular blood vessels remain unaltered.

The muscle atrophy which occurs following nerve sections or lesions of the anterior horn cells (poliomyelitis) is more than a wasting from disuse. It is very rapid in its course, and characteristic changes occur. In addition to the shrinkage of the muscle fibers, degeneration of these cells follows. The cross striations disappear, and a breakdown of the muscle cells ensues. In later stages, the disintegrated muscle cells are replaced by fibrous tissue and fat. Changes also occur in the intramuscular blood vessels. There is an increase in capillaries, and the small intramuscular blood vessels show hypertrophy of the endothelium and an increase in their fibrous structure.

Chor and his co-workers believed that atrophy and degeneration of denervated skeletal muscle are inevitable and then showed that massage did not prevent atrophy up to a period of six weeks; but because of its effect upon the amount of fibrous tissue formed, it did enable the muscles to return to normal more rapidly upon reinnervation.

Langley and Hashimoto studied the effects of massage in denervated muscles of one rabbit. "Firm" massage was given beginning third day postoperative. Treatment was discontinued on the seventh day, because open lesions developed on the limb. Treatment was started again on the eleventh day with "gentler" massage, which was continued until twenty-three days following denervation. They concluded that "at best the effect of the treatment on atrophy was slight" and that an increase in the growth of connective tissue is a possible result of massaging a denervated muscle.

Hartman, Blatz, and Kelborn tested both weights and work capacity of denervated muscles in thirty-seven rabbits. One leg of the animals was given kneading and stroking massage. Both legs were given passive exercise. Treatment was continued for periods varying from seven to one hundred and ninety days. It was found that sixty-two per cent of the massaged muscles were stronger than the controls but not significantly so. Seventeen of the muscles did not agree in function and weight tests. The investigators suggested that the weight of the muscle was not necessarily indicative of the amount of contractile tissue present.

Hartman and Blatz later tested the power of denervated gastrocnemius muscles of sixty rabbits. The muscles on one side were massaged for periods of from two to twenty minutes daily and both legs were given daily passive movement. The muscles were tested at various intervals, ten to fourteen days apart. They concluded that "the treated limb on the whole did not appear to be any better off than the control," that massage was of no value, that there was an invariable decrease in power, with no significant differences between treated muscles and controls.

S. Wright stated that more rigorous proof is required for the claims that muscle wasting is prevented or muscle nutrition improved by massage when unaccompanied by movements. He believed that some local effects are undoubtedly produced in the muscle, that these may be due to chemical agents liberated or expressed into the blood to produce local or general effects, or that some of the metabolites of muscular activity may be liberated by massage. He questioned whether direct mechanical stimulation can produce a direct muscular response in denervated muscle in which reflex reactions are excluded.

Suskind, Hajek, and Hines made studies of denervated gastrocnemius muscles of cats. Two five-minute periods of stroking (effleurage) and kneading (pétrissage) massage were given daily to one limb and the other used as control. Measurements of strength and weight of the muscles were made twenty-eight days after sectioning. These investigators found that "the denervated muscles which received massage were heavier and stronger than their untreated contralateral controls. The effect on muscle weight was slight but statistically significant. . . . Massage . . . served to lessen the gradual loss of contractile strength which occurs in skeletal muscle after denervation."

Wood studied the effects of massage on weights and tensions of the anterior tibial muscle of fourteen dogs. Bilateral sections of sciatic nerves were done, and one leg was given a ten-minute period of stroking and kneading massage daily. The other leg was used as control. The muscles were tested at intervals of from thirteen and a half to thirty-six weeks following denervation. Wood observed that "all anterior tibialis muscles in the treated animals appeared pale and small in bulk as compared to normal anterior tibialis muscles. There was a greater proportion of tendon to total bulk than in normal muscles, and a greater proportion of fatty tissue. It was impossible to distinguish treated from untreated muscle by gross examination. . . . Histological sections from anterior tibialis muscles of treated animals (treated and untreated muscles) showed no marked histological differences." Wood concluded that "massage was not effective in delaying denervation atrophy, as indicated by losses in strength and weight, and by examination of histological sections in experimentally denervated anterior tibial muscles of the dog."

FIBROSIS AND CONTRACTURES

Fibrosis occurs in immobilized, injured, or denervated muscles. A contracture often results. The muscle as a whole becomes shorter than its normal resting length because of the lack of elasticity of the fibrous tissue and the formation of adhesions between layers of connective tissue.

It is possible by massage to apply tension on this fibrous tissue, the objective being to prevent adhesions from forming and to break down small adhesions which have formed. The movements by which this can be accomplished are kneading and friction.

SUMMARY

(1) Massage will not directly increase strength of normal muscle, although as a means to an end it is more effective than rest to promote recovery from fatigue produced by excessive exercise. Theoretically, then, massage makes it possible to do more exercise which will, in turn, increase muscular strength and endurance. This is an important factor in treatment. It would seem logical that massage should be given between periods of exercise when exercise is used to develop muscle strength and endurance.

(2) It cannot be said that massage will increase muscle tone.

(3) Massage may lessen the amount of fibrosis which inevitably develops in immobilized, injured, or denervated muscle.

(4) Massage will not prevent atrophy in denervated muscle. Although a muscle may undergo considerable wasting, if fibrosis is at a minimum and the circulation and nutrition good, a small muscle may have greater power than a muscle of greater weight (this greater weight being due to overgrowth of fibrous tissue which interferes with the function and recovery of remaining innervated muscle fibers).

(5) What one wishes to accomplish by massage is to maintain the muscles in the best possible state of nutrition, flexibility, and vitality so that after recovery from trauma or disease the muscle can function at its maximum.

Effects on the Lungs

Percussive and vibratory massage are used in combination with other measures of chest physical therapy in the prevention and treatment of acute and chronic lung conditions. The few controlled studies on the effects of chest physical therapy do not separate the effects of the various measures. However, clinicians stress the importance of these types of massage in treatment of such conditions as emphysema, bronchiectasis, asthma, atelectasis and pneumonia.

Cyriax (in Licht's *Massage, Manipulation and Traction*[49]) states that percussive techniques, combined with postural drainage, can dislodge mucus and mucopurulent material from the bronchi, and that gravity and vibration help move the secretions from the insensitive periphery of the lung to the area where the cough reflex is beneficially invoked.

Bendixon et al.[5] recommend vibration and percussion with cupped hands with the aim of shaking loose secretions. Percussion is used in cases of "sticky, thick secretions that defy normal coughing efforts."

Cherniack, Cherniack and Naimark[14] feel that the role of physical therapy in the care of patients with acute respiratory failure cannot be overemphasized. While postural drainage is being done to remove secretions "the chest should be pummeled with rapid repetitive strokes and vibrated" with frequent coughing and expectoration of the loosened secretions.

Effects of Massage on Blood

Mitchell stated that, in both health and anemia, the red cell count increased after massage. In anemia, the increase is greatest one hour after treatment. Schneider and

Havens showed that abdominal massage will increase the hemoglobin and red blood cell count in blood taken from the finger at ordinary barometric pressures. Pemberton[62] stated that massage unquestionably increases the hemoglobin and red cells of the circulating blood and that there is a limited but definite increase in the oxygen capacity of the blood after massage. Lucia and Rickard found that massage consisting of gentle but firm stroking of a rabbit's ear at the rate of 25 strokes per minute for five minutes caused a local increase in the blood platelet count.

Bork, Karling and Faust's[9] studies on the effect of whole body massage on serum enzymes in normal persons showed a significant rise in serum GOT, CPK, LDH and MK. They regard whole body massage to be contraindicated for patients with dermatomyositis, especially serious cases, because of these effects.

Effects of Massage on Skin

Little is known about skin metabolism. Therefore, it is difficult to evaluate how this may be affected by massage. Some authorities[44] state that massage produces a direct effect on the superficial layers of the epidermis, that the openings of the sebaceous and sweat glands are freed, and that this, with the improved circulation, directly improves the function of these glands. S. Wright said that sweat secretion is not significantly increased but that sebaceous secretions may be expressed.

According to Rosenthal[20] massage increases the temperature of the skin from 2° to 3°C. He found that neurasthenic persons, under conditions similar to those of tested normal individuals, showed a higher increase in the temperature of the skin, and women showed higher increase than men. He explained the differences by the fact that the entire nervous system, including the vasomotor nerves, is more easily stimulated in neurasthenics than in normal individuals, and in women than in men. The increase in skin temperature may be due to direct mechanical effects and to indirect vasomotor action.

Severini and Venerando found that both superficial and deep massage led to a significant fall in skin temperature at the site of application. Barr and Taslitz found that increased sweating and decreased skin resistance to galvanic current resulted from massage. They found a wide variation in changes in skin temperature in both control and treatment periods and felt they could not infer that massage either increased or decreased skin temperatures.

Clinical observation shows that following massage to a part which has been in a cast for some weeks a definite improvement in the texture and appearance of skin can be noted.

If the skin has become adherent to underlying tissues and scar tissue is formed, friction movements and tension are useful mechanically to loosen the adherent tissues and to soften the scar.

Bodian[7] recommends the use of massage to achieve better cosmetic results following surgery of the eyelid. The modus operandi of the method he describes "seems to be stretching and disruption of excess scar tissue." He has found this massage useful in treating thick scars of the lid, keloid formation, overcorrected ptosis, overcorrected entropism, postoperative ectropism, and shallow fornices.

Effects of Massage on Fatty Tissue

Claims have been made that massage will remove deposits of adipose tissue in various regions of the body. Krusen states that clinical observations will not support this theory and that attempts to reduce local depositions of fat are futile.

Rosenthal[20] investigated this problem experimentally. Vigorous massage was applied to certain areas of the abdominal wall of animals. Microscopic studies made of the massaged and untreated areas showed that there was no change in the fat tissue of the treated areas, although the massage had been severe enough to cause frequent small hemorrhages.

S. Wright and Kalb made similar statements in their studies.

Effects of Massage on Bone

Key and his co-workers conducted an experiment to determine the effects of heat, massage or active exercise upon local atrophy of the bone which is caused by the immobilization of the part. Ten patients with normal lower extremities were used. Both extremities were placed in a cast which was bivalved and removed during treatment. One extremity was used as a control; the other was treated. The massage was given ten minutes, twice daily for six weeks. Roentgenograms were made before and at the end of the experiment, and comparison showed that the atrophy was of practically the same degree in the control extremities as in those which were massaged. They concluded that short periods of heat (five patients), massage (two patients), or active exercise (three patients) had little if any effect on the local atrophy of bone which occurs by immobilization in a plaster of paris cast.

Massage is widely used in the treatment of fractures and is considered beneficial in aiding the repair of the accompanying injuries which occur to the soft tissues. It has not been established that massage aids in the actual healing of the bone. However, in the process of normal bone repair, after fracture, it was the opinion of The Fracture Committee of the American College of Surgeons in 1940 that "The effectiveness and rapidity of growth of tissue are dependent upon efficient circulation in the parts.... Therefore every effort must be made from the beginning to help the efficiency of the circulation."

Mock stated, "Some recent research tends to show that callus is formed along the lines of the new blood vessels formed at the site of fractures, and therefore anything aiding circulation in the area of the fracture *without producing motion of the fragments* should aid in the deposition of callus."

Effects of Massage on Metabolism

Very little recent experimentation has been done on the effects of massage on metabolism, although several studies were made over fifty years ago. Cuthbertson, in 1933, reviewed the literature on this subject and also conducted several experiments of his own at this time. These studies indicate:

(1) There is an increase in the output of urine, especially following abdominal massage.

(2) The excretion of acid is not altered and there is no change in the acid-base equilibrium of the blood.

(3) There is an increased rate of excretion of nitrogen, inorganic phosphorus, and sodium chloride.

(4) In normal persons there is no immediate effect on the basal consumption of oxygen, or on the pulse rate or blood pressure.

Pemberton[60] believed that "in general the studies which have been made suggest broad and general influences may be exerted by massage and that it has no immediate or large effect on general metabolism per se." He agreed with Rosenthal that its cumulative effect on various metabolic processes lies in its influence on the circulation of the parts concerned.

Effects of Massage on Viscera

ABDOMINAL VISCERA

There is little information in recent literature on the effects of massage upon the abdominal viscera.

Mennell believed that the heavy abdominal massage which was formerly taught apparently was given for mechanical effect, and that this was an error arising from lack of comprehension of the object in view. He pointed out that the slightest tap on an exposed intestine of a frog causes instant spasm of that portion and also cardiac inhibition and that the effect of manipulation upon involuntary muscle of the intestines can be observed during abdominal surgery—excessive handling may result in overstimulation and temporary paralysis of the unstriped muscle.

Mennell's opinions about the true effects of abdominal massage follow. To empty the contents of the small intestine mechanically is obviously impossible, he believed. Any action of massage on the intestines is almost, if not entirely, reflex in response to the mechanical stimulation of pressure. This stimulation can increase peristalsis and, thereby, hasten the emptying of the contents. He pointed out that some portions of the large intestine are quite constant in their relationship to the abdominal wall, and thus the direction of the passage of the contents in the duodenum, the ascending and descending colon, and the iliac colon can be followed.

Beard and Wood were convinced that massage of the abdomen by use of the techniques of kneading and deep stroking as described under "local massage of the abdomen" (pages 142–143) is effective in increasing peristaltic action to promote evacuation of flatus and feces from the large intestine. These procedures may be carried out by the patient while he is seated on the stool.

The contents of the abdomen, with the exception of the duodenum and fixed portions of the colon, may easily be displaced or glide away from any pressure exerted on the abdominal wall, making it impossible to exert any mechanical effect of massage.

Mennell believed that although it may be possible to secure a definite mechanical effect from massage in the treatment of some of the abdominal organs (e.g., prostate), the effects are probably due to a reflex reaction to mechanical stimulation.

He said that reflexly it may be possible also to produce contraction of the unstriped muscle of the spleen, but physiologically it is difficult to explain any beneficial effect.

To expect any benefit from "shaking up the liver," as had been recommended by earlier writers on massage, is wrong, according to Mennell, although abdominal massage may aid the portal circulation and, thus, all the functions of the liver.

Massage for treatment of the pancreas has been suggested by some writers; Mennell thought it possible that this organ can be influenced reflexly, but it would seem probable that it is only the indirect effect produced by improving the general vascular tone.

The gallbladder being a hollow organ is, according to Mennell, amenable to the mechanical effects of massage.

Because knowledge of the effects of massage on the abdominal viscera is quite limited, and until more specific information is available, it would seem unwise for the physical therapist to apply any type of abdominal massage except that which will affect the muscles of the abdominal wall and possibly indirectly influence the circulation, and also, through reflex response to pressure, stimulate activity of the involuntary muscle of the intestines.

Special techniques are required for massage of specific organs, and they should be applied only by the physician or the physical therapist especially trained by him in these techniques. (Because of the possible harm which might result from abdominal massage, it should not be included in a general massage without first obtaining specific directions from the physician.)

OTHER VISCERAL ORGANS

Mennell questioned the use of massage for the kidneys. Although he noted that by kneading the kidney it is possible during cystoscopy to see urine pass from the ureter into the bladder, he doubted that this is clinically practical.

Massage for stimulation of the heart is used as an emergency treatment. When an abdominal incision has been made, the surgeon may massage the heart either by compressing the heart between the diaphragm and the ribs or by incising the diaphragm and directly grasping the heart. Mennell knew of no direct action upon the heart as a result of the usual externally applied massage movements.

In 1960, Kouwenhoven and co-workers reported a seventy per cent permanent survival rate of patients with cardiac arrest who were given closed-chest cardiac massage (see Appendix, pages 151–152).

Psychological Effects of Massage

Most persons are familiar with the soothing effect of gentle massage, even when there is no pathology or physical disability present.

The therapist's concentrated attention to the patient, combined with the pleasant physical sensation which results from the massage, seem to establish a close and trusting personal relationship in which the patient often reveals to the therapist problems, worries, and facts about his health which he has thought too minor to tell the doctor.

The therapist acts as a listener who guards all such revealed information as confidential. He is careful to see that the patient does not become too dependent in the relationship, and encourages the patient to reveal to his physician those facts which the doctor should know.

Negative psychological effects can result from massage treatment. The time and attention required for massage may exaggerate in a patient's mind the seriousness of his disability. Mennell warned, "It is easier to rub a disability into a patient's mind than it is to rub it out of his limb." Care must be taken to reassure the anxious patient and to correct his misinterpretation of the reason for his treatment.

General massage is frequently prescribed as a temporary form of treatment while the physician is awaiting the development of the specific treatment of a patient. The knowledge that something is being done for him often aids in relieving the patient's anxiety regarding his illness.

SUMMARY

It is evident that the studies on the effects of massage reviewed in this chapter have in many instances omitted any mention of the details of the massage applications, so that conclusions drawn by the experimenters and clinicians had to be stated in quite general terms.

Many references on the clinical use of massage state that "massage does (or does not) . . ."; "massage will (or will not) . . ."; "massage should (or should not) be used for . . ."; "massage is indicated (or contraindicated) in the treatment of . . .", —absolute statements which are seldom based upon knowledge or consideration of the effects of specific types, amounts, or sequences of massage movements applied to specific tissues.

This situation will not change until (and unless) many competent, controlled, clinical and laboratory studies are done which evaluate the many possible combinations of the various components of massage. These studies must be correlated with up-to-date physiological and pathological concepts. With the many new instruments and techniques for biological research now available, individual and cooperative-group studies by physicians, physical therapists, physiologists, and engineers can provide clinicians, both doctors and therapists, with more knowledge about many aspects of applied massage, so that treatment can be prescribed and given on a scientific rather than an empiric basis.

chapter 5

technique

REQUIREMENTS FOR MASSAGE

Thoughtful concentration is necessary for the intelligent application of massage.

Basic Technique

The following points are essential for good technique in all massage:
a. To maintain evenness of rhythm.
b. To establish correct rate of movement.
c. To keep hands flexible so as to fit the contour of the area.
d. To maintain proper postural stance.
e. To regulate pressure according to the kind of tissues being treated and the purpose of the treatment.

These essentials must be observed in all massage movements and are more important for good technique than the various specific movements that may constitute so called "systems" of massage.

RHYTHM

Evenness of rhythm has been discussed in the description of massage movements (see Chapter 3, page 42). Its importance in good massage technique is again emphasized. It must be used in all massage movements.

RATE OF MOVEMENT

The rate of massage movements has also been discussed in the description of the movements (see Chapter 3, pages 38, 42). For the reasons previously stated, a "slow" rate should be established and followed throughout all massage movements except those of percussion and vibration.

FLEXIBILITY OF HANDS

Certain persons seem to possess a natural ability to relax their hands and to move them rhythmically, and they will learn the technique of massage more readily than others. However, anyone who conscientiously spends sufficient time in practice will learn contact and rhythm, and acquire good technique.

STANCE

Controlled relaxation of the hands can be obtained only if the posture of the physical therapist is one that permits controlled relaxation and free movement of the arms.

The so-called standing "fall-out" position will make such relaxation possible. Standing at the side of the table, facing the patient's head, the physical therapist should advance the foot farthest from the table, keeping the other foot back (Fig. 17).

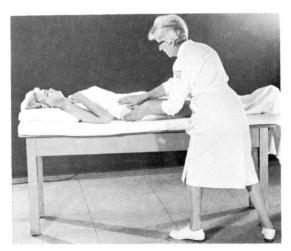

Figure 17

A backward and forward swaying movement made with the knees and ankles bent will then permit the arms and hands to be used over a large area with comparatively little movement at the hips or spine. Both feet should be kept in contact with the floor at all times to maintain balance. This swaying makes it possible to perform long stroking movements rhythmically and smoothly, allows proper relaxation of arms and hands, and avoids unnecessary fatigue (experienced from performing massage when standing in a strained, stooped position). It also utilizes the weight of the body in regulating the amount of pressure applied. Swaying is unnecessary in applying movements of small amplitude, and unnecessary movement of the body should be avoided, for it may be annoying to the patient and cause unnecessary fatigue to the physical therapist.

PRESSURE AND CONTACT OF HANDS

All massage must be given directly on the skin. Only the therapist's sense of touch and the thoughtful and intelligent realization of this sense can develop the judgment necessary to regulate pressure correctly. Long and careful practice is required to develop this ability.

As has been stated before, the pressure need not be heavy, if the muscles are relaxed, and should be such as will not cause injury to the delicate structures under treatment or produce pain. The only exception to this is when compression movements are used to stretch adherent and shortened tissues. In this instance, slight injury to the adherent tissues may be necessary in order to loosen them, and some pain may be produced if shortened tissues are stretched. This pain must be transient and not continue for a period longer than one-half hour after the part is placed at rest. If pain continues for a longer period, it is evidence of an overdose of treatment.

In all palmar movements the entire palm, or as much thereof as is necessary to fit the contour of the area to be massaged, must be in close contact. Obviously this is necessary if the purpose of the massage is to be attained. The greater the area that the hand contacts, the greater is the amount of tissue influenced by the same amount of pressure. This is simply illustrated by attempting to squeeze fluid out of a soft tube.

In movements performed with the thumb or other digits, the distal phalanx should be in slight hyperextension, so that as much as possible of the distal phalanx is in contact and so that contact with the fingernails is prevented. The remainder of the hand should be in light contact while movements are performed with the thumb.

Equipment

The most essential equipment for massage is a pair of well-trained hands directed by an intelligent mind. Other equipment should consist of:
  a. A firm table, its height appropriate for correct posture of the therapist.
  b. A mattress firm and sufficiently thick for the patient's comfort.
  c. Adequate amount of linen and pillows.
  d. Lubricant.

TABLE

The height of the massage table should make it unnecessary for the physical therapist to stoop or reach up to perform the movements; the average height is 28 inches. The width (24 to 26 inches) should be sufficient to allow the patient to turn from side to side easily but not so wide that the physical therapist must either move the patient closer to the edge of the table or be out of proper stance. The table should have a drawer or shelf to accommodate needed linen and cold cream, unless a bedside table or shelf is provided, and should be accessible from both sides and both ends.

MATTRESS

The mattress should be not more than three inches in thickness to facilitate the application of the massage movements. (A mattress cover should be used for protection.) The mattress should be smoothly and firmly covered with a sheet.

LINEN AND PILLOWS

The patient should be covered with a sheet, and a light blanket if necessary for warmth. Small towels, for removing excess lubricant, and bath towels, if necessary for covering local parts, as well as a sufficient number of pillows for support to the patient, should be close at hand.

The bedding should always be kept neatly arranged. To avoid soiling the bed linen by contact with the lubricant, a towel may be placed under each area as it is treated, and a towel may be folded over the edge of the sheet and blanket where they are turned back to expose the section to be massaged.

LUBRICANT

Some type of lubricant should be used in nearly all massage movements to avoid irritation of the patient's skin and to insure smooth contact. Cold cream is preferable to liquid oils because of the convenience of application. The cream should be of a type which is slightly absorbed by the skin and yet not so oily that a large amount is left on the skin after the massage is completed; the United States Pharmacopeia (U.S.P.) formula is one that has been found suitable. Only a sufficient amount to allow smooth gliding over the skin should be used, as too much lubricant will prevent a firm grasp of the tissues and will leave an excess amount on the patient's skin. The amount will depend upon the dryness of the patient's skin and of the hands of the physical therapist. Experience will make it possible for the physical therapist to develop the sense of touch necessary to choose the correct amount to be used. The correct amount for one area should be put on both palms and applied to the area with the first stroking movement. Any excess amount at the completion of the massage to each area should be removed with a soft towel by gentle rubbing in the centripetal direction.

In some instances, a fine unscented talcum powder or French chalk may be substituted for cold cream as a medium to prevent irritation of the patient's skin, but usually it does not permit as satisfactory a grasping of the tissues as does a cream lubricant.

To obtain the firm contact with the skin that is necessary to apply friction movements, it is important that no lubricant be used. In using friction movements over dry, scaly scar tissue the friction should be applied without the medium, and when the friction is completed a small amount of lubricant should be applied to the area with stroking movements.

If the patient's skin and the palms of the physical therapist are dry, it is often possible to use stroking or kneading movements of small amplitude quite satisfactorily without a medium of any sort.

Position of the Patient

The patient should be placed in a comfortable position, with sufficient support of the area to be treated to insure relaxation of all muscles. All clothing should be removed from the part to be treated. No tight clothing should be allowed to restrict circulation in the proximal areas of an extremity which is being treated (for example, a rolled-up trouser leg when a knee, leg, or foot is being treated). Care should be taken to keep the patient warm, and all parts of the body which are not being massaged should be covered by a sheet or towels.

The part being treated should be in a position to either eliminate resistance to gravity or permit gravity to assist in the venous flow of the blood, the flow of lymph, and the elimination of mucus and other fluids from the lungs, or to avoid pressure on a traumatized area of the body. This can best be accomplished by placing the patient in a recumbent position with adequate support provided by the use of pillows. Support must be given to the entire part being treated (extremity or trunk) to avoid strain on joints.

When the patient is in the supine position, a pillow may be placed under the head and a small pillow or rolled bath towel should be placed under the knees. When the patient is in the prone position, a pillow should be placed under the abdomen. A small pillow or rolled bath towel under the ankles will prevent extreme plantar flexion at the ankle joint. This may also be accomplished by placing the patient so that his feet extend over the end of the table. There should be no pillow under the head. When the patient is sidelying, as is sometimes necessary because of pain, the need to avoid pressure after trauma or surgery, the presence of bulky casts or bandages, or respiratory problems, pillows should be used wherever necessary to give support to head, anterior and posterior aspects of the trunk, and both upper and lower extremities of the side on which the patient is not lying.

The patient should under most circumstances be recumbent during massage to any area of the body. An exception may be made in treating the hand or forearm, when no edema or disturbance of the circulation is present and when the muscles of the arm and shoulder are functioning normally. Under these conditions the patient may be seated at a small table of a height to give comfortable support at the elbow, with the forearm and hand resting on the table. The therapist should be seated opposite on a stool or chair which permits free movement of the arms (Fig. 18).

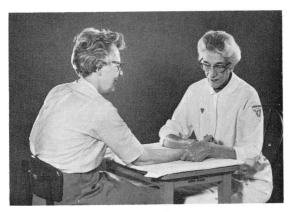

Figure 18

Another exception could be made when massaging shoulder and upper back and neck muscles, if the prone position is too painful for the patient to assume. In this case the patient should sit in a chair facing the table and lean forward from the hips; the trunk, shoulders, neck, and head should be well supported by pillows and the forearms and hands should rest on the table on either side of the pillow support. The therapist should stand behind the patient, or slightly to one side, to give the massage (Fig. 19).

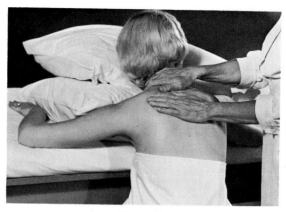

Figure 19

The therapist should never sit on a patient's bed or table nor support an extremity on his lap.

Routine of Treatment

All preparation for a massage treatment and the routine of the treatment should be carried out quietly and systematically. The bedding should be neat at all times. Any appearance of hurry before, during, or after the treatment should be avoided. (If efficiency is practiced in planning and performing the day's work and punctuality is observed in keeping appointments, under usual circumstances hurry should not be necessary.)

Each movement should be purposeful. There should be no aimless wandering of the hands over any area. To administer massage effectively, the therapist should give thoughtful attention to the condition of the tissues as determined by the contact of his hands and should select the type of movement that will accomplish the desired results. Continuity of contact should be observed when a change is made from one movement to another. Any break in contact and replacement of the hands produces a stimulus to the sensory nerve endings in the skin.

Superficial stroking, for its relaxing effect, should be the introductory movement and may be used to apply the lubricant to the area to be treated. Deep stroking, starting with light pressure, should follow. This will permit the therapist to evaluate the condition of the tissues in the area. The amount of pressure in the deep stroking may be increased gradually to the maximum amount suitable for the firmness of the tissue. Kneading and stroking movements may be alternated. Kneading may follow the deep stroking to influence further the blood and lymph flow and to promote absorption of substances within the tissues. The alternation of these movements may be continued until the desired effect has been obtained, finishing with the deep stroking and, finally, superficial stroking.

Friction movements should be followed by stroking or kneading movements to assist the circulation, to aid in repair if adhesions have been loosened, and to relieve any pain that may have been produced. Care must be used not to apply friction for too long a period over one area, thus causing unnecessary injury and undue pain.

If edema exists in an extremity, the treatment should begin with the proximal portion. The treatment of the distal segment or segments should follow, with a return to the proximal segment at intervals and for the completion of the treatment. Unless the circulation is improved in the proximal portion first, any attempt to lessen the edema in more distal segments will be quite ineffective; it will be like trying to empty a bottle with the stopper still in place.

All massage movements should be performed slowly and rhythmically, with careful attention to pressure, contact, and all details of administration of the treatment.

GENERAL MASSAGE

Massage applied to the entire body is usually termed "general" massage. Massage cannot be a substitute for exercise in the attempt to restore function. However, since massage improves the circulation of the blood and lymph, in this respect it is similar in effect to exercise. In certain circumstances, therefore, when the normal active exercise of the body is prohibited and if the existing pathology is not a contraindication, massage is useful. In cases that require a long period of confinement to bed, a daily massage of the entire body will aid materially in assisting the general circulation and bringing a sense of comfort and relaxation to the patient. In elderly people, general massage may substitute for some of their former muscular activity.

As Pemberton stated, general massage may be productive of fatigue. A feeling of mild lassitude by the patient, and a desire for rest immediately following a general massage, is indicative of a successful treatment, and for this reason the patient should rest one to one and a half hours following treatment. Real fatigue should be avoided, and if the patient is not refreshed after a period of rest the duration of the treatment has been too long or the technique of the treatment has been too vigorous.

To accomplish the relaxation and sedation usually desired in general massage, there must be a smooth uninterrupted change from one type of movement to another, and a definite rhythm must be carried out in all movements.

Certain adaptations of the Swedish type of movement seem to be best suited for this form of massage. These movements are performed on an entire segment of each extremity without special attention being paid to any certain muscle or muscle group. The type of massage that does definitely follow muscle groups and specific muscles is more effective in the treatment of local injury or diseased areas and will be described later.

The routine of a general massage should be such that the patient is not required to move or turn from side to side any more than is necessary. The therapist also should change his position as little as possible, and all his movements should be efficient and quiet. The following order of movements will facilitate such a program:

1. The patient is supine with a pillow under his head.

(a) The therapist stands at the right side of the patient and massages the right thigh and leg.

(b) He then moves to the foot of the table and massages the right foot.

(c) He then moves to the left side of the patient and massages the left thigh and left leg.

(d) He then moves to the foot of the table and massages the left foot.

(e) He then moves again to the left side of the patient and massages the left arm, forearm, and hand.

(f) He then moves to the right side of the patient and massages the right arm, forearm, and hand, the chest, and the abdomen. A small pillow may be substituted for the usual one under the head during massage to the chest. This allows the therapist's hands to move smoothly around to the back of the neck.

2. The patient turns to the prone position and the treatment is concluded with massage to the back. (The therapist does not have to change his position for this part of the treatment.)

Because it requires smoothness in movement, relaxation of the hands to allow good contact to the contour of the part, and rhythm of the movements general massage should be the first massage taught to students. Techniques of the contact and rhythm established in this type of massage will be carried through to all massage movements. This requires long and faithful practice, until these skills in massage become instinctive. The therapist can then concentrate on selecting movements that will produce the specific effects desired.

Technique for General Massage

The following outline of technique is the authors' modification of a Swedish system of massage which is well adapted to a general massage. The position of the therapist is as indicated in each section. The patient is supine except for massage to the back.

RIGHT THIGH

The therapist stands at the side of the table on the patient's right.

(1) Superficial Stroking.

Both hands reach around the thigh, covering it as much as possible, and stroke from the anterior superior spine of the ilium to the knee (Figs. 20, 21, 22, 23).
[Do this movement four times.]

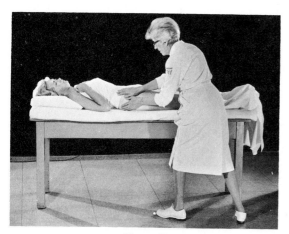

Figure 20

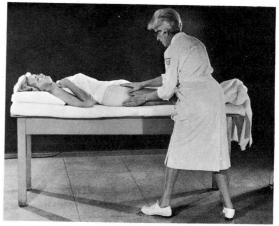

Figure 21

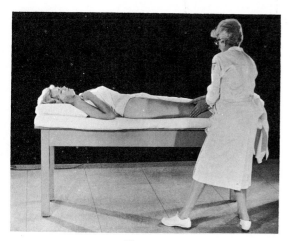

Figure 22

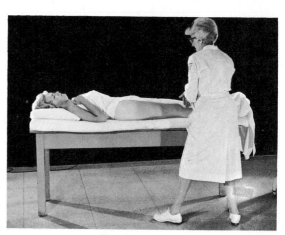

Figure 23

(2) Palmar Kneading to the Quadriceps.

The ulnar border of the right hand is placed below the patella, with the thumb placed on the lateral border and the fingers on the medial border of the patella.

The left hand picks up the distal portion of the muscle above the patella (Fig. 24).

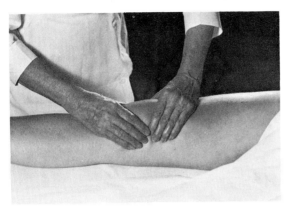

Figure 24

The right hand strokes over the patella toward the left hand, with the ulnar border keeping firm contact in the upward pressure. The muscle is grasped between the thumb and the fingers and is held firmly into the palm. The palmar surface of the fingers of the left hand pulls the muscles laterally as the surface of the abducted right thumb and palm simultaneously pushes the tissues medially. Then the surface of the palm and abducted thumb of the left hand push the muscles medially as the palmar surface of the fingers of the right hand pulls the tissues laterally. Progression from the distal to the proximal part of the quadriceps is accomplished with a gliding of the hands on the "pull" stroke of the kneading movement (Fig. 25).

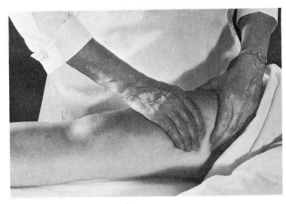

Figure 25

This is not a pinching type of movement. The thumb and fingers of each hand are kept in the same relationship to each other during the entire movement. The "push" and "pull" are accomplished chiefly by flexion and extension of the arms at shoulders and elbows.

As the origin of the muscle is approached, the left hand is removed and the right hand gently "squeezes out" at the origin of the muscle (Fig. 26) and returns to the lower border of the patella with a superficial stroke (Fig. 27).

[Do this movement three times.]

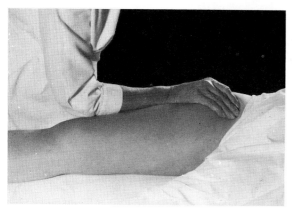

Figure 26

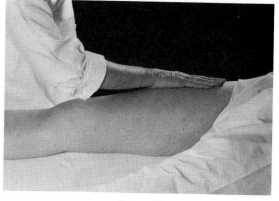

Figure 27

(3) Palmar Kneading to the Posterior Surface of the
Thigh.

The hip and knee are slightly flexed and the thigh slightly rotated externally. Both hands reach across the medial surface of the thigh, grasp the flexors at the knee (Fig. 28), and perform the same type of movement as was done on the quadriceps except that the hands are held more transversely to the muscles (Fig. 29). The movement is terminated a few inches below the hip joint. The left hand is removed; it crosses over the right hand and grasps the muscles above the knee (Fig. 30), and the right hand returns along the medial surface of the thigh with a superficial stroke.
[Do this movement three times.]

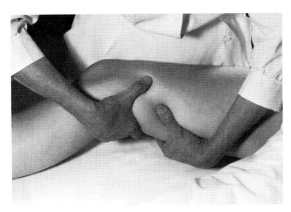

Figure 28

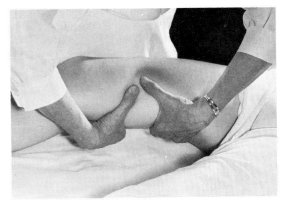

Figure 29

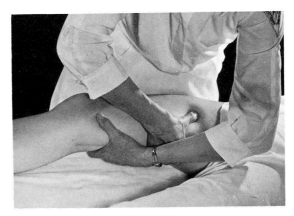

Figure 30

(4) Alternate Palmar Kneading.

Both hands grasp around the upper portion of the thigh (Fig. 31); the hands alternately roll the muscles between the palms with firm pressure upward (Fig. 32), progressing to the knee. Both hands return to the starting position with a deep stroke—see (5) just below.

[Do this movement three times.]

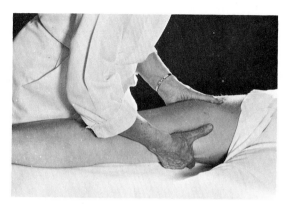

Figure 31   **Figure 32**

(5) Deep Stroking.

Both hands grasp around the thigh just above the knee joint, with the thumbs abducted and the fingers held together. Finger tips of opposing hands are in contact with each other on the posterior surface. With firm pressure of the entire palmar surface, the hands stroke upward to the upper portion of the thigh, then return to the knee with a superficial stroke.

[Do this movement three times.]

RIGHT LEG AND KNEE

The therapist stands at the side of the table on the patient's right.

(1) Superficial Stroking.

Both hands stroke from the knee joint to the ankle joint, covering the entire surface of the leg (Figs. 33, 34, 35).
[Do this movement three times.]

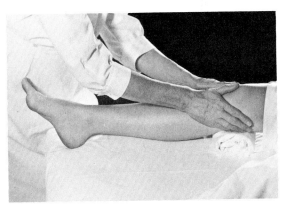

Figure 33

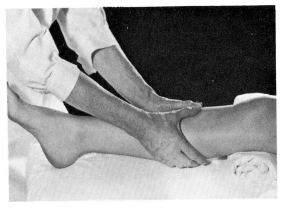

Figure 34

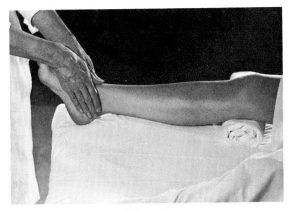

Figure 35

*(2) Thumb Kneading Over the Tibialis Anterior and
Underlying Muscles.*

    The distal phalanx of each thumb is placed in firm contact at the origin of the
muscle; the rest of the hand rests lightly on the surface of the leg (Fig. 36). The
thumbs move alternately in circles, with pressure upward and outward. The hands
glide to the more distal adjacent area as each circle is made. The movement progresses in this manner (Fig. 37) to the ankle joint (Fig. 38). The hands return to the
starting position, with the thumbs giving deep stroking and the rest of the hand maintaining light contact.

[Do this movement two times.]

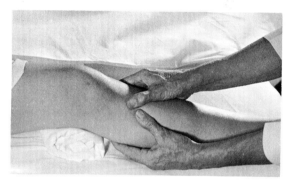

Figure 36

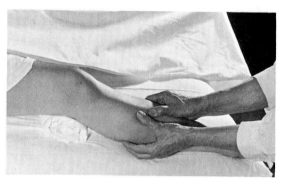

Figure 37

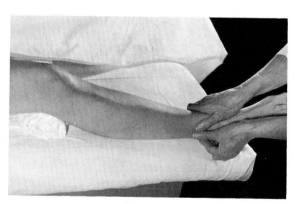

Figure 38

(3) Palmar Kneading to the Calf Muscles.

The right hand supports the slightly flexed knee joint at the medial border.

The left hand grasps the muscle group just below the knee, and the muscles are pulled toward the lateral border of the leg, with the palmar surface of the fingers exerting pressure (Fig. 39). Then the palmar surface of the abducted thumb and thenar eminence pushes the muscles upward and toward the medial border of the leg (Fig. 40). The fingers then glide distally and these movements are repeated, until the hand reaches the ankle (Fig. 41). The hand then returns to the knee with a deep stroke over the muscles.

[Do this movement three times.]

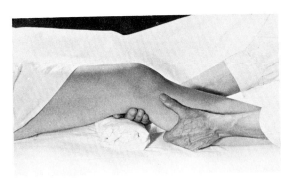

Figure 39

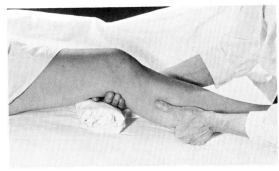

Figure 40

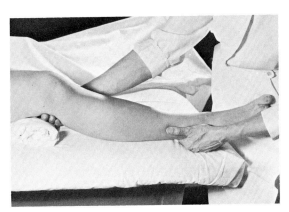

Figure 41

Change hands: support the knee with the left hand, and repeat the procedure with the right hand.

[Do this movement three times.]

(4) Alternate Palmar Kneading.

Both hands grasp around the muscles at the knee and alternately roll the muscles between the palms with firm pressure upward, working to the ankle. The hands are returned to the knee with a deep stroke over the muscles. (This is the technique used in alternate palmar kneading of the thigh. See page 70.)

[Do this movement three times.]

(5) Palmar Stroking Around the Patella.

The heels of both hands are placed at the lower border of the patella; the palmar surface of the distal phalanges of the fingers is in contact with the skin above the proximal border of the patella (Fig. 42). The thenar eminences of both hands stroke firmly around the patella in a circular movement by allowing the fingers to flex while the tips are kept in light contact (Fig. 43). The heels of the hands return to the beginning position with a superficial stroke distally, allowing the thumbs to glide lightly over the patella.

[Do this movement four times.]

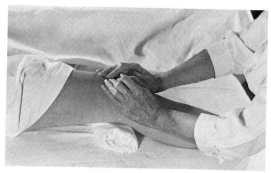

Figure 42

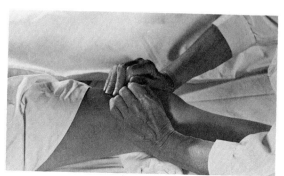

Figure 43

(6) Digital Stroking Over the Popliteal Space.

The finger tips of both hands are placed together at the distal border of the popliteal space; then they stroke firmly to the proximal border and return to the starting position with a superficial stroke.

[Do this movement four times.]

(7) Deep Stroking, with Both Hands, to the Entire Leg.

[Do this movement three times.]

RIGHT FOOT

The therapist stands at the foot of the table, facing the patient.

(1) Superficial Stroking over the Dorsum of the Foot.

The palmar surface of the right hand on the sole of the foot gives support, and the left hand strokes from the ankle (Fig. 44) to the end of the toes (Fig. 45), alternating over the lateral and the medial dorsal surfaces.
[Do this movement two times.]

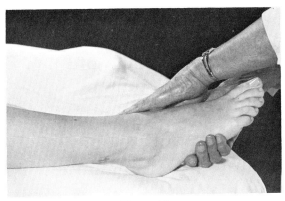

Figure 44

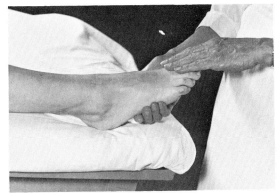

Figure 45

(2) Thumb Kneading over the Dorsum of the Foot.

The distal phalanx of each thumb is placed in firm contact on the medial surface of the foot, distal to the medial malleolus, and the fingers rest on the plantar surface of the foot (Fig. 46). Thumb kneading, as described for tibialis anterior, is performed, progressing from the ankle to the metatarsal phalangeal joints. The thumbs return to position with deep stroking over the same area. The kneading is repeated in successive lateral sections until the entire dorsum of the foot is covered (Fig. 47).
[Do this movement two times.]

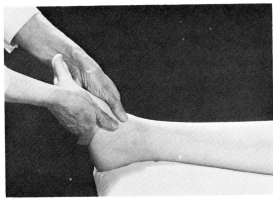

Figure 46

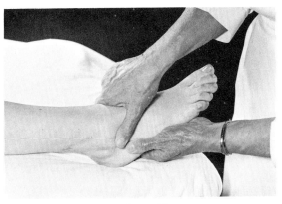

Figure 47

(3) Thumb Stroking to the Plantar Surface of the Foot.

The thumbs are placed at the base of the toes, the right at the inner border, the left at the outer border of the plantar surface. The fingers rest lightly on the dorsum of the foot (Fig. 48). The thumbs stroke firmly in opposite directions from the borders of the foot, passing in the center (Fig. 49). The stroking progresses from the base of the toes to the heel. The movement is performed chiefly by abduction and adduction of the arms at the shoulder. The thumbs are removed, and the fingers keep contact and return to the starting position with a superficial stroke.
[Do this movement two times.]

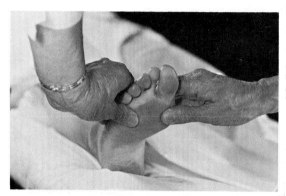

Figure 48

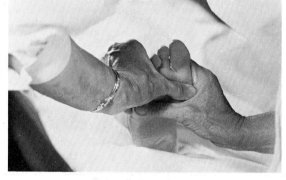

Figure 49

(4) Palmar Stroking to the Plantar Surface of the Foot.

The therapist pivots to face across the end of the table. The left hand on the dorsum of the foot gives support. The ulnar border of the right hand is placed firmly on the plantar surface at the base of the toes (the hand is in supination) (Fig. 50). As the hand strokes firmly down to the heel with deep pressure, it is pronated and made to fit well into the arch (Fig. 51), finishing with the palm flat on the table.
[Do this movement four times.]

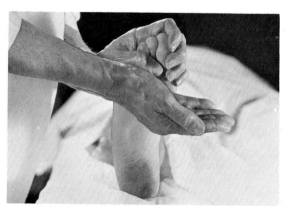

Figure 50

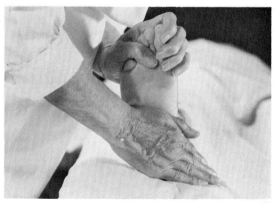

Figure 51

(5) Digital Stroking around the Malleoli.

The therapist pivots back to face the head of the table. Both hands are placed on the dorsum of the foot, with the tips of the fingers at the base of the toes, the index fingers together, and the thumbs crossed (Fig. 52). The fingers perform deep stroking toward the ankle joint with firm pressure. At the ankle the hands separate; fingers of the left hand stroke around the lateral malleolus as the fingers of the right hand stroke around the medial malleolus (Fig. 53). The palmar surfaces of the fingers keep firm contact, fitting into the contour of the foot as they circle back to the dorsum of the foot and return to the base with a superficial stroke.

[Do this movement four times.]

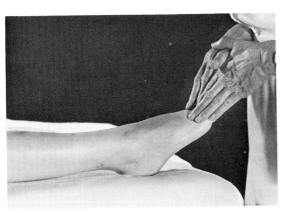

Figure 52

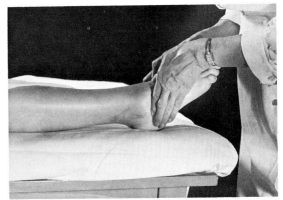

Figure 53

(6) Digital Stroking of the Achilles Tendon.

The wrists are flexed and the radial sides of the index fingers stroke firmly upward on each side of the tendon (Fig. 54). Without losing contact, the hands turn so that the ulnar side of the little fingers can stroke lightly downward to the heel (Fig. 55).

[Do this movement four times.]

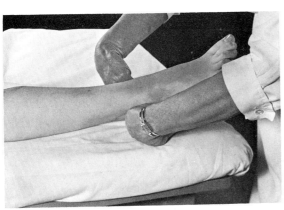

Figure 54

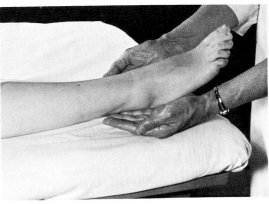

Figure 55

(7) Deep Stroking to the Leg and Thigh.

The therapist returns from the foot to the side of the table, and the hands glide into position for deep stroking of the leg. Both hands perform deep stroking to the entire leg and thigh and return to the foot with a superficial stroke.
[Do this movement three times.]

(8) Superficial Stroking to the Entire Thigh, Leg, and Foot.

[Do this movement four times.]

LEFT THIGH, LEG, AND FOOT

The physical therapist stands at the left side of the patient. The movements are the same as those performed on the right extremity, except that the right hand is substituted for the left hand and the left hand is substituted for the right hand.

LEFT ARM, FOREARM, AND HAND

The therapist continues to stand at the left side of the table, but in a position which will enable him to massage the upper extremity easily.

(1) Superficial Stroking.

Both hands stroke from the shoulder (Fig. 56) to the finger tips (Fig. 57).
[Do this movement four times.]

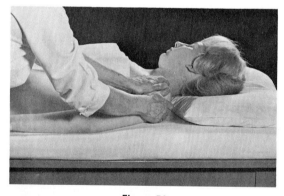

Figure 56

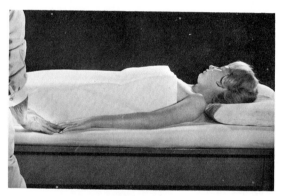

Figure 57

(2) Alternate Palmar Stroking over the Deltoid.

The hands are placed just distal to the borders of the deltoid muscle (Fig. 58). The right hand, in firm contact, strokes upward over the posterior half of the deltoid (Fig. 59). As it returns with a superficial stroke, the left hand strokes upward over the anterior half of the deltoid (Fig. 60). As it returns with a superficial stroke, the right hand starts its second stroke (Fig. 61).

[Do this movement ten times.]

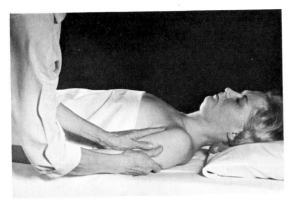

Figure 58

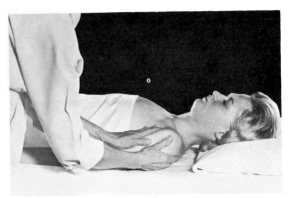

Figure 59

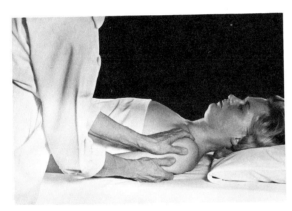

Figure 60

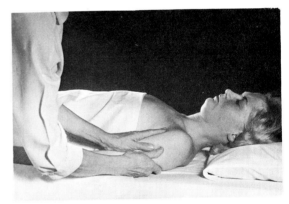

Figure 61

(3) Thumb Kneading to the Upper Extremity.

The procedure is similar to movements described for the tibialis anterior group (see p. 72). However, the entire surface of the limb is covered in three sections—anterior, lateral, and posterior surfaces (Fig. 62). Kneading is done from the shoulder to the wrist, and the hands return with a deep stroke from the wrist to the shoulder. [Do this movement two times.]

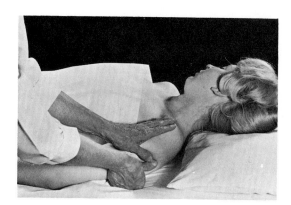

Figure 62

(4) Palmar Kneading to the Arm and Forearm.

The right hand does palmar kneading as described for the leg, while the therapist supports the patient's arm with his left hand, for kneading to the arm (Fig. 63), and then allows the arm to rest on the table while his supporting hand passes to the wrist, giving support at the wrist while the forearm is kneaded (Fig. 64). Tissues of the lateral part of the arm and forearm are kneaded by the right hand. The right hand returns to the shoulder and the left hand returns to the elbow with a superficial stroke, and kneading of the arm and forearm is repeated.

At the end of the second kneading, the left hand returns to the shoulder and the right hand returns to the elbow to support the arm in slight external rotation and forearm in supination. Kneading of medial tissues is then done by the left hand as the right hand supports. At the end of the second left-hand kneading, both hands return to the shoulder with a deep stroke (similar to that done on leg and thigh). [Do this movement three times with each hand.]

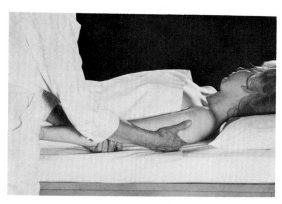

Figure 63

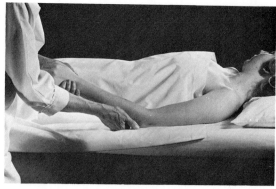

Figure 64

(5) Alternate Palmar Kneading.

This movement is performed on the upper extremity in the same manner as described for the leg (see page 73), working from the shoulder to the wrist (Figs. 65, 66).

[Do this movement three times.]

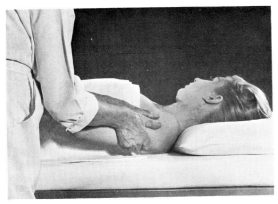

Figure 65

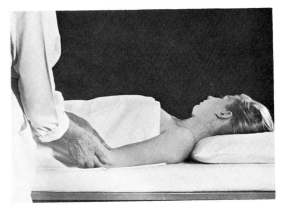

Figure 66

On the last repeat, the hands do not return to the shoulder with a deep stroke but remain at the wrist, to begin thumb kneading to the dorsum of the hand.

(6) Thumb Kneading to the Dorsum of the Hand.

Thumb kneading is performed, working from the wrist to the metacarpo-phalangeal joint in each metacarpal space (Fig. 67), as described in thumb kneading to the dorsum of the foot (see page 75).

[Do this movement two times.]

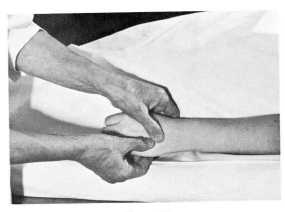

Figure 67

*(7) Thumb Stroking to the Palmar Surface of the
Metacarpophalangeal Joints.*

The patient's hand is held in supination and supported on the fingers of both hands, with the left thumb at the medial border and the right thumb at the lateral border (Fig. 68); the thumbs stroke toward and past each other (Fig. 69) with firm pressure and return with light pressure, as described for the plantar surface of the foot (see page 76).

[Do this movement four times.]

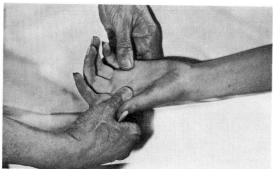

Figure 68

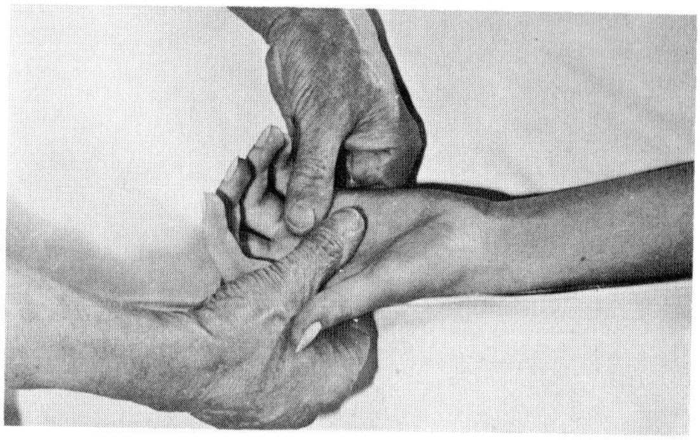

Figure 69

*(8) Thumb Stroking over the Thenar and Hypothenar
Eminences.*

The patient's hand is held in supination, supported on the fingers of both hands, with the left thumb on the hypothenar eminence and the right thumb on the thenar eminence (Fig. 70). The thumbs stroke in alternation toward the wrist with firm pressure and return with light pressure.

[Do this movement four times.]

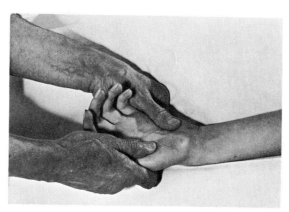

Figure 70

(9) Thumb Kneading to the Thumb and Fingers.

The hand is held in pronation and supported in the palm of the left hand. The right thumb, beginning at the metacarpophalangeal joint (Fig. 71), kneads on a small area of the medial aspect of the little finger with firm pressure in the centripetal direction, passes lightly over the dorsum of the finger, and kneads on the lateral aspect; the thumb then moves lightly back over the dorsum of the finger and repeats the movement in the area just distal; this procedure is continued to the tip of the finger (Fig. 72). The thumb and the first finger then stroke firmly back to the base of the finger. The entire movement is done twice on each finger. The thumb is massaged in the same manner, except that the right hand gives support while movements are performed with the left (Fig. 73).

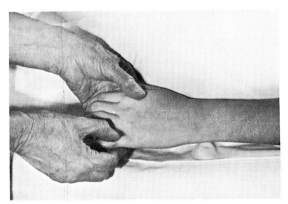

Figure 71

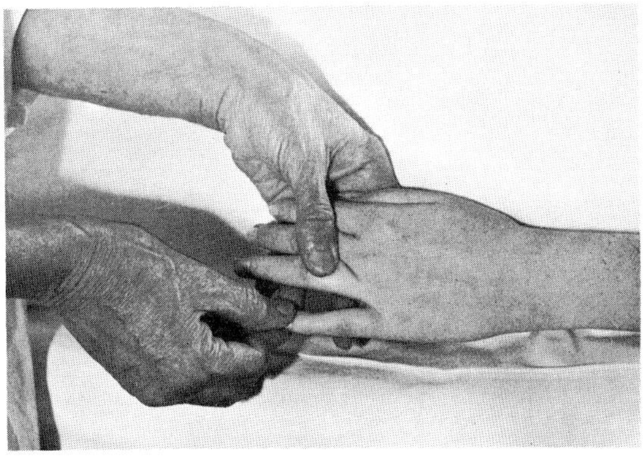

Figure 72

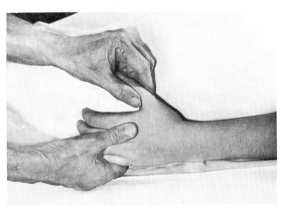

Figure 73

(10) Deep Stroking.

Both hands stroke firmly upward from the wrist to the shoulder and return with a superficial stroke.

[Do this movement three times.]

After the third deep stroke, the superficial return stroke becomes the start of superficial stroking.

(11) Superficial Stroking.

Both hands stroke from the shoulder to the finger tips.
[Do this movement four times.]

RIGHT ARM, FOREARM, AND HAND

The therapist walks around the foot of the table and stands at the patient's right side near the right hand.

The movements are performed on the right upper extremity in the same manner as those on the left, except that the right hand is substituted for the left hand and the left hand is substituted for the right.

CHEST

The therapist stands at the side of the table on the patient's right.

(1) Superficial Stroking.

The hands alternately stroke from the shoulders to the sternum. The right hand starts from the patient's right shoulder and, as it finishes the stroke at the sternum, the left hand starts the stroke from the left shoulder so that contact is not broken. The right hand starts again as the left hand finishes its stroke (Fig. 74).
[Do this movement four times.]

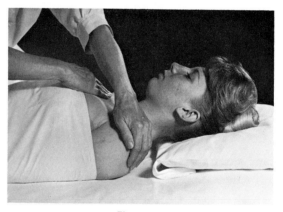

Figure 74

*(2) Deep Stroking over the Shoulder and
Around the Neck.*

Both hands, with the thumbs adducted, are placed with the finger tips at the lower end of the sternum (Fig. 75). The hands stroke simultaneously, the right hand passing lightly upward, then laterally and around the left shoulder joint, and the left hand passing lightly upward, then laterally and around the right shoulder joint (Fig. 76). Both hands continue the movement, stroking toward the midline of the body along the upper fibers of the trapezius.

(a) After the fingers meet at the lower cervical spine, the hands then stroke deeply over the top of the shoulder and return to the starting position at the sternum (Fig. 77).

Repeat the first part of the movement, as described, to (a). Then (b), after fingers meet at lower cervical spine, the hands stroke around the neck, firmly drawing the muscles forward (Fig. 78). Pressure lightens as the hands stroke over the anterior surface of the neck and return to the starting position at the sternum.

[Do this movement two times, alternating (a) and (b).]

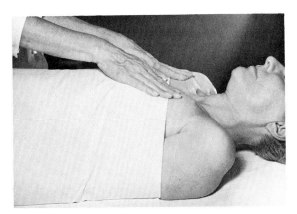

Figure 75

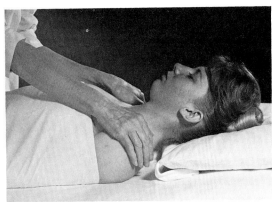

Figure 76

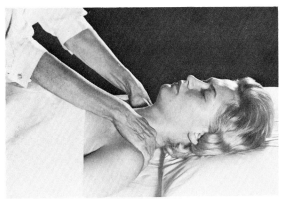

Figure 77

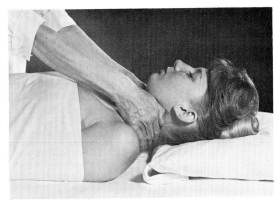

Figure 78

*(3) Digital Kneading from the Sternum to
the Shoulder.*

The finger tips of the right hand are placed at the sternum over the upper fibers of the left pectoralis major, and the left hand is placed over the right hand to reinforce it (Fig. 79). The kneading is done with the finger tips, in small clockwise circles, with light pressure on the upward and outward part of the circle and firm pressure in the downward and inward part of the circle. Four circles are made, each succeeding one in an area nearer to the shoulder. As the finger tips reach the shoulder joint, the palm strokes around the joint (Fig. 80), and the entire hand returns, and strokes deeply as it returns to the sternum.
[Do this movement three times on the left side.]

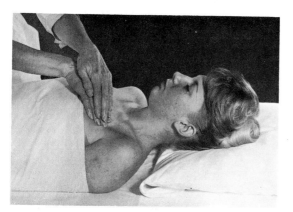

Figure 79

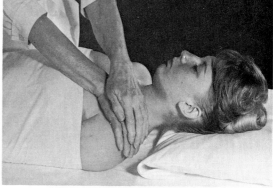

Figure 80

With the hands in the same position, the movement is done on the right side, in counterclockwise circles (Fig. 81).
[Do this movement three times on the right side.]

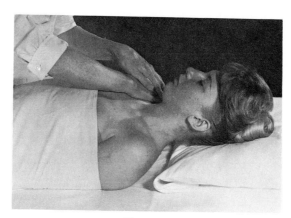

Figure 81

*(4) Alternate Deep Stroking from the
Shoulder to the Sternum.*

The hands are in the same position as in Fig. 79. With the entire palmar surface, the right hand strokes lightly to the left shoulder joint. The palm then strokes around the joint and returns to the sternum, with firm pressure (as in the previous movement). Repeat this movement on the right side.

[Do this alternate stroking four times.]

(5) Digital Stroking around the Neck.

The hands start in the same position as in Fig. 79. The right hand strokes over the top of the left shoulder and in toward the midline of the body. When the finger tips reach the lower cervical spine, they stroke upward until the palm is in contact with the neck. The hand then draws the muscles forward with firm pressure (Fig. 82), exerts light pressure over the anterior surface of the neck and the clavicle, and returns to the starting position. The stroking is then done the same way on the right side (Fig. 83).
[Do this alternate stroking four times.]

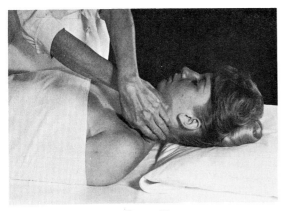

Figure 82

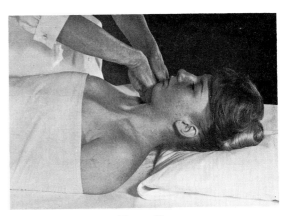

Figure 83

(6) Deep Stroking over the Jugular Veins.

With the thumbs widely abducted, the palmar surface of the fingers of the right hand is placed on the left side of the neck, and that of the left hand is placed on the right side of the neck, with the borders of the index fingers at the lower tips of the ears (Fig. 84). The hands stroke firmly downward to the base of the neck as the forearms are pronated and the arms are abducted (Fig. 85). The thumbs must not make any contact. With gradually lessening pressure, the hands continue the stroke out to and off the shoulder tips (Fig. 86).

[Do this movement four times.]

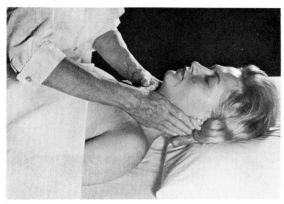 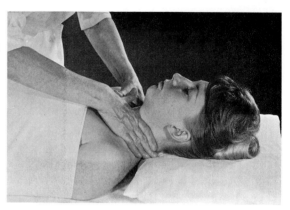

Figure 84   *Figure 85*

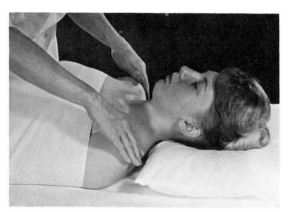

Figure 86

(7) Deep Stroking.

Repeat (2) (see page 85) but gradually reduce the pressure with each stroke, until the last stroke is done as superficial stroking.

ABDOMEN

The therapist stands at the side of the table on the patient's right. The patient's knees are flexed and supported with a pillow.

(1) Superficial Stroking.

The right hand, with the thumb widely abducted, is placed over the lower border of the left ribs:the left hand is similarly placed over the lower border of the right ribs. Both hands stroke simultaneously to the symphysis pubis, covering the entire abdomen. The hands are lifted off at the end of the sroke and returned to the starting position without contact with the skin.

[Do this movement four times.]

(2) Deep Stroking.

The finger tips of both hands are placed side by side at the symphysis pubis. The right hand strokes lightly outward to the left anterior superior spine, while the left strokes to the right anterior superior spine (Fig. 87). Both hands continue stroking above, and following the crest of, the ilium around to the back until they meet at the upper lumbar spine. The palms then stroke forward with firm pressure around the waistline (Fig. 88) and over the abdomen to the symphysis pubis. (The purpose of this movement is to manipulate the abdominal musculature, not to exert pressure upon the abdominal contents.)

[Do this movement four times.]

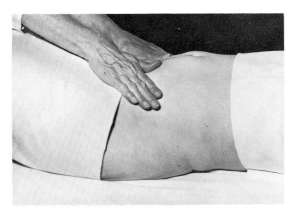

Figure 87

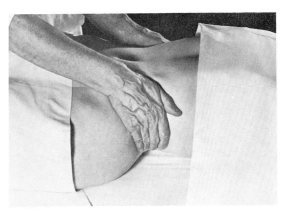

Figure 88

(3) Deep Stroking over the Upper Abdomen.

The right hand is placed so that the fingers lie over the lower anterior border of the left ribs and the palm is at the base of the sternum; the left hand is placed over the right hand for reinforcement (Fig. 89). The right hand strokes lightly in the lateral direction over the ribs, then down over the upper abdominal muscles (Fig. 90), and then returns to the starting position with firm pressure over the upper abdomen.
[Do this movement four times on the left side.]

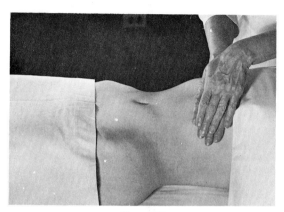

Figure 89

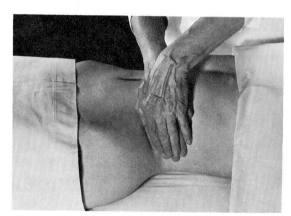

Figure 90

Next, place the right hand with the finger tips at the base of the sternum and the palm over the lower anterior border of the right ribs (Fig. 91). Follow the above procedure on the right side (Fig. 92). In order to have the right palm in good contact on this side, the right wrist must be in full extension at the start (Fig. 91) of the stroke.
[Do this movement four times on the right side.]

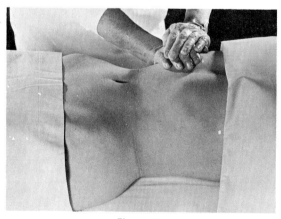

Figure 91

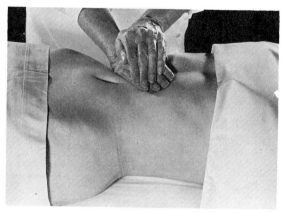

Figure 92

(4) Palmar Kneading over the Colon.

The right hand is placed over the lower right quadrant of the abdomen, so that the ulnar border of the hand lies along the pubic bone and just medial to the anterior superior spine of the ilium (Fig. 93).

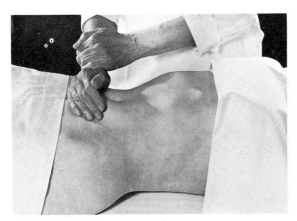

Figure 93

The left hand reinforces the right hand. The ulnar border of the right hand lifts up the tissues in a "scooping" sort of movement performed by pressure with the ulnar border of the hand, rolling the hand over to the thenar border as the palm is pushed toward the finger tips which are kept in contact with the skin all during this "scooping" movement (Fig 94). The finger tips are then moved to a more proximal point on the ascending colon as the hand rolls back onto its ulnar border and the movement is repeated. Using this movement, the massage progresses over the abdomen, covering the areas of the ascending, the transverse, and the descending colon. The movement is changed slightly over the descending colon so that the firm pressure is with the thenar eminence of the palm and in a distal direction. The movement is completed with a firm stroke downward over the lower part of the area of the descending colon (Fig. 95) and the hand passes lightly over the lower abdomen to the area of the lower border of the ascending colon.

[Do this movement three times.]

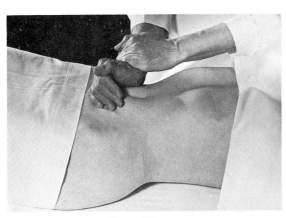

Figure 94

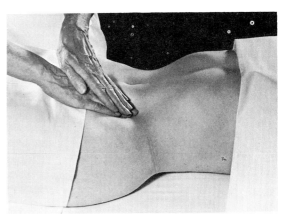

Figure 95

(5) Deep Stroking over the Colon.

The finger tips of the right hand are placed at the lower border of the area of the ascending colon: the left hand reinforces the right (Fig. 96). The finger tips stroke firmly upward over the area of the ascending colon, across the area of the transverse colon (Fig. 97), and downward over the area of the descending colon (Fig. 95), then lightly over the lower abdomen to the starting point.

[Do this movement six times.]

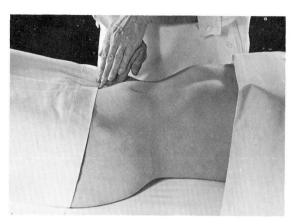
Figure 96

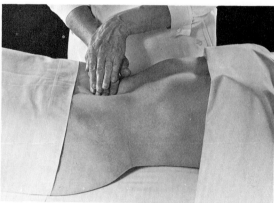
Figure 97

(6) Alternate Palmar Kneading over the Entire Abdomen.

At the right side of the abdomen, both hands, with the thumbs abducted, grasp the tissues, and by alternate flexion and extension at the elbows and the shoulders progress across the abdomen with a kneading movement (Fig. 98). Both hands return together to the right side with a superficial stroke.

[Do this movement four times.]

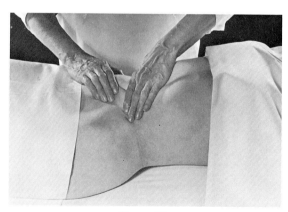
Figure 98

(7) Deep Stroking.

Repeat (2) (see page 89), gradually reducing the pressure to superficial stroking.

BACK AND HIPS

The therapist stands at the side of the table on the patient's left. The patient is prone, with a pillow under the abdomen and one under the ankles. The patient's head may be turned to either side for comfort.

(1) Superficial Stroking.

The right hand is placed over the right shoulder and the left hand is placed over the left shoulder, with the thumbs just lateral to the spinous processes of the first cervical vertebra (Fig. 99). Both hands, with thumbs abducted, stroke simultaneously to the sacrum, covering as much of the back as possible (Fig. 100). The hands return in the air to the starting position.
[Do this movement four times.]

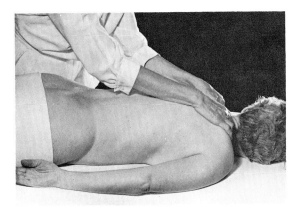
Figure 99

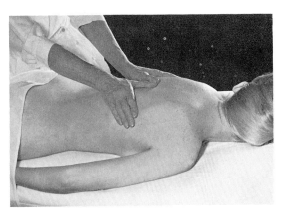
Figure 100

At the end of the fourth stroke, the hands keep contact so they are in position to start deep palmar stroking.

(2) Deep Palmar Stroking.

The fingers of both hands start the deep stroke at the lower border of the sacrum; the thumbs are crossed for reinforcement (Fig. 101), and the hands stroke upward on each side of the spinous processes with firm pressure.

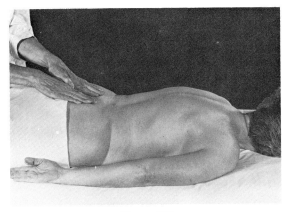
Figure 101

(a) The hands separate at the neck and stroke over the top of the shoulder, as the thumbs stroke up to the first cervical vertebra on both sides of the spinous processes (Fig. 102). The hands then stroke back, drawing the muscles back also, until the finger tips are at the top of the shoulder (Fig. 103). At the same time, the thumbs stroke down on both sides of the cervical vertebrae. The hands, with thumbs adducted, then stroke laterally to the shoulder joint (Fig. 104) and down the sides of the back to the waist-line, and then toward the midline (Fig. 105) and down until the finger tips are at the lower border of the sacrum. (Thumbs cross to reinforce as the hands start the downward stroke to the sacrum.)

(b) The hands stroke upward and over the shoulder as in (a) Fig. 102) and return the stroke downward until the finger tips are even with the axilla (Fig. 106), then pass laterally and stroke to the sacrum as in (a).

(c) The hands stroke upward and over the shoulder as in (a), return the stroke downward until the wrists are at the waistline (Fig. 107), then pass laterally and stroke to the sacrum as in (a).

(d) The hands stroke upward and over the shoulder as in (a), then return the stroke downward until the finger tips are at the waistline (Fig. 108), then pass laterally and stroke to the sacrum as in (a).

(e) The hands stroke upward as in (a) and return the stroke over the shoulder and then downward, with the hands spread to cover the entire back, and return to the sacrum (Fig. 109).

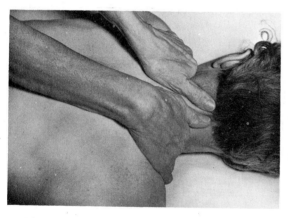

Figure 102

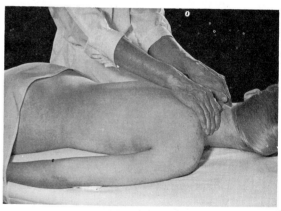

Figure 103

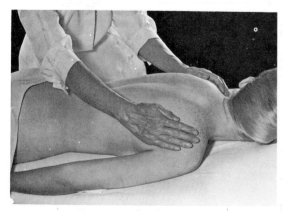

Figure 104

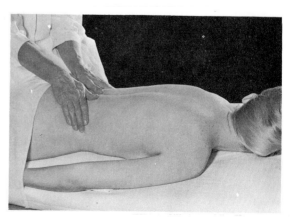

Figure 105

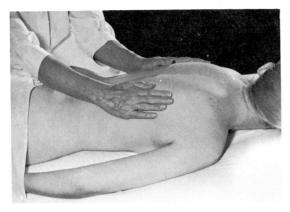

Figure 106

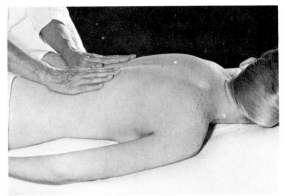

Figure 107

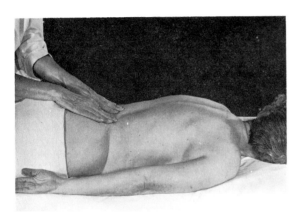

Figure 108

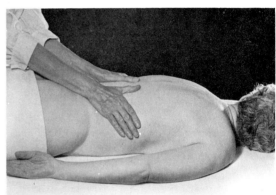

Figure 109

*(3) Digital Kneading over the Upper Fibers
of the Trapezii.*

The finger tips of the right hand, reinforced with the left hand, are placed at the upper cervical region of the right trapezius (Fig. 110). They knead in small clockwise circles, exerting heavier pressure when making the last of each circle. The kneading progresses to the acromion process (Fig. 111). The fingers return to the starting position with a superficial stroke.

[Do this movement three times.]

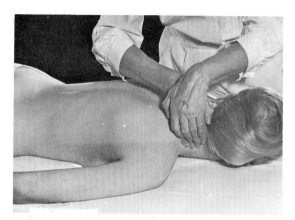

Figure 110

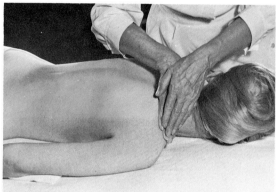

Figure 111

The left side is kneaded in the same manner, except that circles are made counterclockwise.

[Do this movement three times.]

*(4) Digital Stroking over the Upper Fibers
of the Trapezii.*

The thumbs are placed on the borders of the trapezii, lateral to the spinous processes of the upper cervical vertebrae and with the palms of the hands over the tops of the shoulders. Both hands stroke firmly to the acromia, picking up the muscles as the thumbs reach the lower cervical region (Fig. 112). The hands return with a superficial stroke.

[Do this movement four times.]

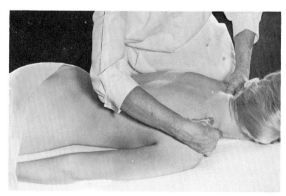

Figure 112

(5) Palmar Kneading over the Scapular Region.

The right hand, reinforced by the left hand, is placed with the palm above the spine of the right scapula and the thumb just lateral to the spinous processes of the upper dorsal vertebrae. The palm kneads in a clockwise circle over the upper scapular region (Fig. 113), then glides to make a second circle over the lateral border of the scapula, a third circle over the lower angle of the scapula, and a fourth over the medial border of the scapula.

[Do this movement three times.]

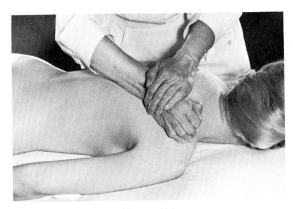

Figure 113

Transition is made from one side to the other with no break in contact; the hand glides with a superficial stroke.

To massage the left scapular region, the right hand is placed with the palm above the spine of the left scapula and the ulnar border of the hand just lateral to the spinous processes of the upper dorsal vertebrae. The kneading is done in the same manner as for the right side, except that the circles are made counterclockwise.

[Do this movement three times.]

*(6) Alternate Palmar Kneading over (to) the
Dorsal and Lumbar Regions.*

Both hands are placed at the left side of the upper dorsal region. The left hand strokes across to the lateral border of the right dorsal region with firm pressure (Fig. 114) and, as this hand returns to the left side, the right hand strokes across to the right side. The muscles are kneaded by the alternate movement between the hands. As the right hand returns, the left hand again strokes to the right side. These strokes are repeated, the hands alternating in direction and progressing to the lower border of the lumbar region (Fig. 115). Before the left hand completes the stroke at the lower lumbar area, the right hand is removed and is placed on the upper dorsal region to start the entire kneading movement again.

[Do this movement four times.]

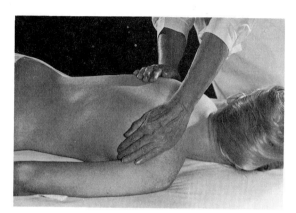

Figure 114

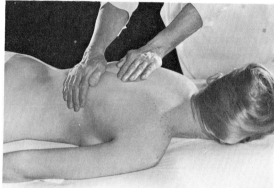

Figure 115

(7) Palmar Stroking over the Lumbar Region.

The right hand, reinforced by the left, is placed over the lower ribs on the right side, the fingers extending along the ribs (Fig. 116). The hand strokes lightly from the spine to the lateral lumbar region of the right side and returns below the ribs, stroking toward the spine with firm pressure (Fig. 117).

[Do this movement four times.]

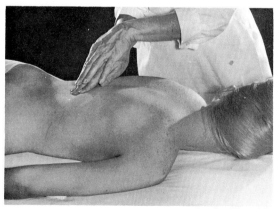

Figure 116

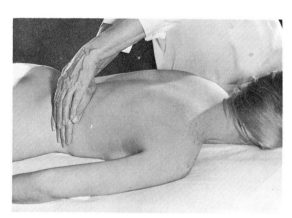

Figure 117

The left side is massaged in the same manner as the right, except that the right hand is placed with the finger tips at the spine for the initial stroke.
[Do this movement four times.]

(8) Thumb Kneading over the Sacrum.

The thumbs of both hands are placed at the upper border of the sacrum, with the palms in contact with the back just above the iliac crest (Fig. 118). The thumbs knead alternately, in small circles, with pressure upward, progressing to the lower border of the sacrum. The thumbs stroke upward with firm pressure for the return.
[Do this movement four times.]

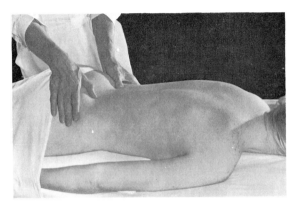

Figure 118

(9) Alternate Palmar Kneading to the Buttocks.

The ulnar border of the right hand is placed at the right gluteal fold, and the ulnar border of the left hand is placed in the area of the origin of the glutei so that the hands can grasp the muscles (Fig. 119) to knead in an alternating movement similar to that described for the quadriceps. Pressure is applied so as to avoid separation of the buttocks.
[Do this movement two times.]

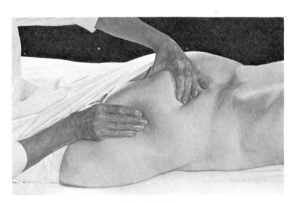

Figure 119

The left buttock is massaged in the same manner as the right.
[Do this movement two times.]

(10) Deep Kneading to the Buttocks.

The left hand supports the muscle, or the left hand may reinforce the right hand, as the right hand does deep kneading over the right buttock (Fig. 120) in the same manner as for kneading over the colon, except that the heel of the hand exerts firm pressure toward the midline throughout the movement, to avoid separation of the buttocks.

[Do this movement two times.]

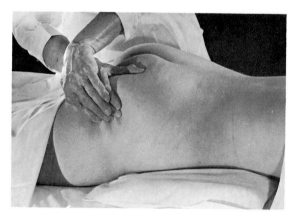

Figure 120

The left buttock is kneaded in the same manner as the right.
[Do this movement two times.]

(11) Alternate Palmar Kneading over the Entire Back.

This movement is the same as in (6) (see page 98) beginning at the upper scapular region and continuing over the entire back.
[Do this movement four times.]

(12) Digital Kneading to the Erector Spinae.

The distal phalanges of the first and second fingers of both hands are placed just lateral to the spinous processes at the lower cervical region, and the distal phalanx of each thumb is placed an inch or two below the finger tips. (This relative position of fingers and thumb is maintained for each hand throughout the movement.) The fingers of the right hand, with firm pressure, draw a portion of the muscle downward; simultaneously the left thumb, with firm pressure, presses a portion of the muscle upward (Fig. 121) then the right thumb presses a portion upward as the fingers of the left hand draw a portion of the muscle downward. Progression from one area to the next is accomplished by a gliding of the fingers during the period of firm pressure, while the thumb of the same hand superficially strokes the area to be covered next. (This kneading of the tissues between the thumb of one hand and the fingers of the other is produced by alternate flexion and extension at the elbows and the shoulders.) The kneading is continued to the sacrum.
[This movement is not repeated. The hands break contact before starting the next movement.]

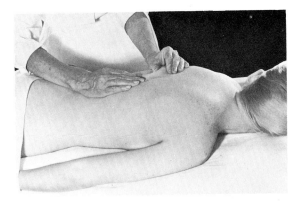

Figure 121

(13) Palmar Stroking to the Erector Spinae.

The entire palm of the right hand is placed over the center of the spine at the cervical region and moves with a superficial stroke to the sacrum. As the right hand approaches the end of the stroke (Fig. 122), the left hand starts another superficial stroke. The right hand returns in the air (Fig. 123).
[Do this movement four times.]

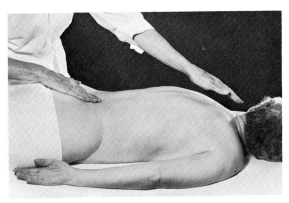
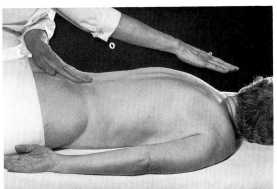
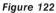

Figure 122   *Figure 123*

(14) Deep Palmar Stroking.

Repeat (2) on pages 93–94 gradually reducing the pressure to superficial stroking.

The number of times indicated for each movement in the technique for general massage is the approximate number required to give a general massage within one hour's time, at the rate of speed established for the movements (see pages 38, 42, Chapter 3). This must not be interpreted to mean that all general massage must be given for exactly one hour or that in all instances every movement in every area must be performed exactly the number of times mentioned. Massage may be contraindicated in certain areas. If the physician so directs, that area should be omitted from the treatment. This is particularly true of the abdomen; therefore it is wise for the therapist to inquire if the abdomen is to be included in the treatment. All massage treatment must be administered according to the prescription for each individual patient and all factors of dosage, as previously stated, must be considered in each treatment.

Technique for Facial Massage

Facial massage may be added to a general massage. Patients with insomnia frequently respond to it particularly well, and it is a useful sedative in the treatment of headache.

The movements are over a small area and should be gentle, so that it is not necessary to use a lubricant. The hands should be washed and thoroughly dried. A small amount of fine talcum powder may be used if the skin is moist from perspiration.

The technique for facial massage that follows is a type recommended for sedation in the treatment of headache and insomnia. If general massage has not been given, the treatment should include the chest and upper back movements as given in general massage.

The patient should be in the recumbent position, with the head supported on a small pillow. The physical therapist stands at the side of the table on the patient's right, facing the patient.

All movements are performed with both hands in unison, with the exception of the thumb kneading over the nose.

FACE

(1) Superficial Stroking.

(a) The palms are placed side by side on the forehead, with the thenar eminences on either side of the midline; the fingers are slightly flexed to fit over the head, with the finger tips resting lightly on the top of the head (Fig. 124).

The palms stroke to the lateral borders of the forehead (Fig. 125) and return to the starting position by moving through the air while the hands pivot on the finger tips.

[Do this movement two times.]

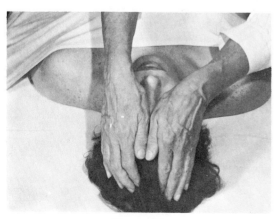

Figure 124

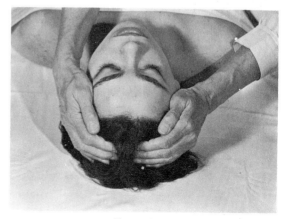

Figure 125

(1) Superficial Stroking—Continued.

(b) The movements are the same as in (a) except that the finger tips rest at the hairline so that the palms are placed over the cheeks (Figs. 126, 127)
[Do this movement two times.]

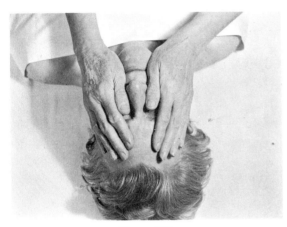

Figure 126

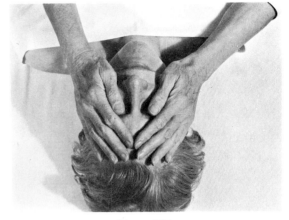

Figure 127

(c) The finger tips glide lightly from the hairline to the temples. The thumbs are placed together at the center of the chin (Fig. 128). They stroke laterally along the border of the mandible to the tip of the ear (Fig. 129) and return to the chin through the air.
[Do this movement two times.]

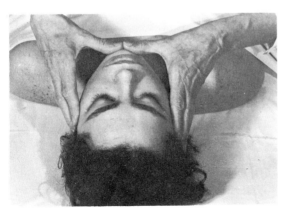

Figure 128

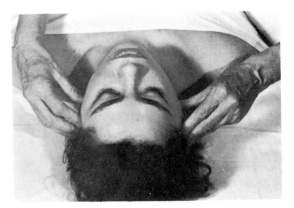

Figure 129

(d) The movements are the same as in (c) except that the thumbs start *under* the chin and stroke under the jaw to the tip of the ear.
[Do this movement two times.]

(2) Circular Thumb Kneading to the Forehead.

The finger tips of each hand keep contact at the temple, and the thumbs are placed together at the center of the lower border of the forehead (Fig. 130). The thumbs knead simultaneously in small circles (Fig. 131), continuing up to the hairline. They return in the air to the lower border of the forehead at more lateral areas and repeat the movements, until the entire forehead is covered.
[Do this movement two times.]

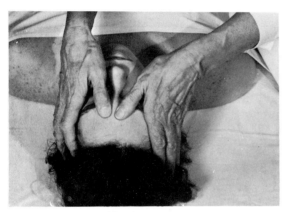

Figure 130

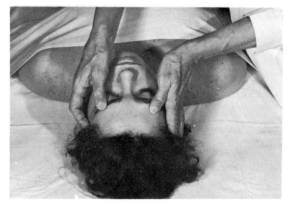

Figure 131

(3) Deep Stroking to the Forehead.

The finger tips of each hand are kept in contact at the temples, and the palms are placed with the radial borders together on the forehead (Fig. 132). The palms stroke laterally from the midline with firm pressure (Fig. 133) and return in the air.
[Do this movement three times.]

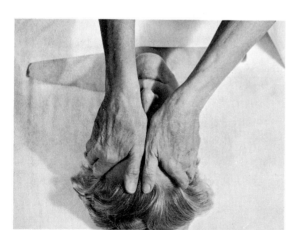

Figure 132

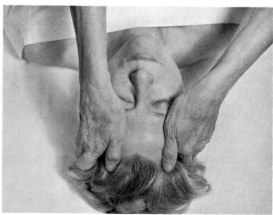

Figure 133

(4) Alternate Thumb Kneading to the Nose.

The finger tips are kept in contact at the temples, and the distal phalanges of the thumbs are placed at the tip of the nose (Fig. 134). Alternate thumb kneading is done on the sides of the nose, up to the bridge. The thumbs pause with firm pressure in the hollows formed by the bridge of the nose and the medial part of the supra-orbital ridge (Fig. 135) and then return in the air.
[Do this movement three times.]
At the end of the third kneading, the thumbs keep contact at the hollows, ready to start the next movement.

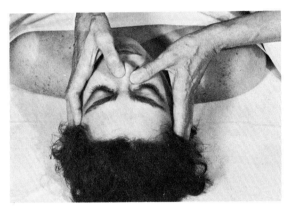

Figure 134

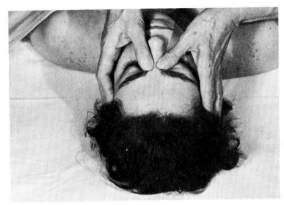

Figure 135

(5) Deep Stroking to the Supra-orbital Ridge.

Continuing from (4) without breaking contact, the thumbs stroke outward with firm pressure over the supra-orbital ridge (Fig. 136) and return in the air.
[Do this movement four times.]

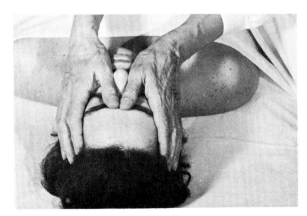

Figure 136

(6) Deep Stroking to the Infra-orbital Ridge.

The hands remain in the same position as for (5), and the thumbs stroke over the infra-orbital ridge (Fig. 137) and return in the air.

[Do this movement four times.]

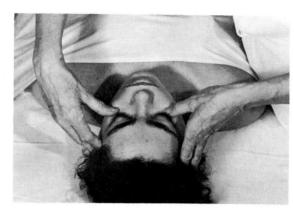

Figure 137

(7) Digital Kneading from the Temple to the Cervical Spine.

(a) The thumbs remain in the air, and the finger tips [without breaking the contact they have maintained at the temples in (2), (3), (4), (5), and (6)] simultaneously knead in small circles, starting at the temple (Fig. 138) and, following the hairline, continuing back of the ears until the fingers meet at the cervical spine (Fig. 139).

(b) Without breaking contact, the fingers stroke with firm pressure down the cervical spine to the seventh cervical vertebra. The thumbs then make contact with the anterior borders of the trapezii, and the stroking is continued with the thumbs and fingers over the upper fibers of the trapezii (Fig. 141) (gradually reducing pressure) to the tips of the shoulders. The hands return to the temples in the air.

[Do this movement two times.]

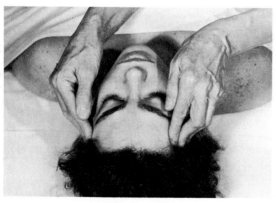

Figure 138

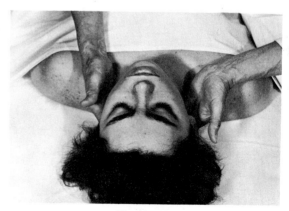

Figure 139

(8) Digital Kneading from the Temple to the Shoulder.

The finger tips knead in small circles from the temple (Fig. 140), passing in front of the ear to the mastoid process and continuing over the sternocleidomastoid and the upper fibers of the trapezius (Fig. 141) to the tip of the shoulder. The hands return in the air.

[Do this movement two times.]

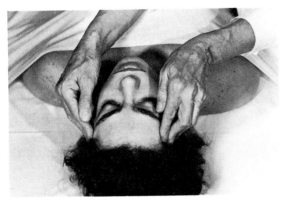

Figure 140

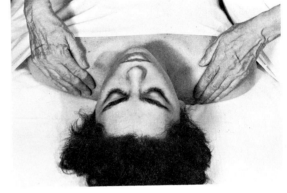

Figure 141

(9) Deep Stroking over the Jugular Veins.

This movement is the same as that described in (6) under Massage of the Chest (see page 88).

[Do this movement four times.]

(10) Palmar Kneading to the Cheeks.

The finger tips rest lightly on the forehead while the palms rest lightly on the cheeks and knead in circles—three times in a forward direction (Fig. 142), three times in a backward direction (Fig. 143). The palms do not move over the skin but with gentle pressure move the tissues over the bony surface.

[Do this movement two times.]

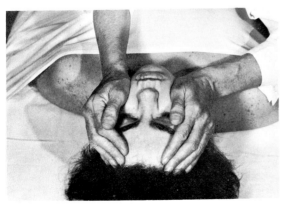

Figure 142

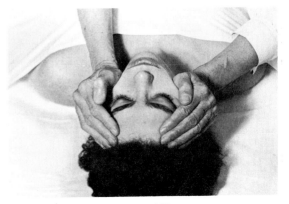

Figure 143

(11) Thumb Kneading to the Chin and the Jaw.

The finger tips glide lightly to make contact below the ears. The thumbs are placed together at the center of the lower border of the chin (Fig. 144) and knead simultaneously in small circles upward to the lower lip, return with superficial stroking, and knead over more lateral areas of the chin. They continue this kneading over the mandible to the tip of the ear (Fig. 145).

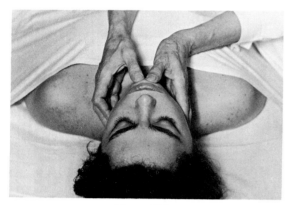

Figure 144

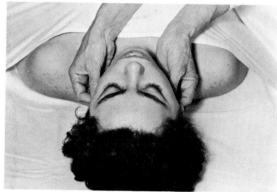

Figure 145

(12) Deep Stroking to the Chin and the Jaw.

Keeping the fingers in contact, the thumbs return to the chin as at the start of (11). They then stroke with firm pressure from the chin (Fig. 146) to the tip of the ear and return in the air.

[Do this movement three times.]

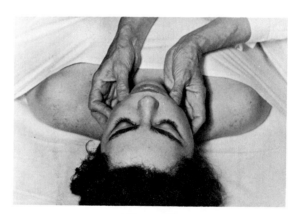

Figure 146

(13) Deep Stroking over the Jugular Veins.

Without breaking contact after (12), repeat the procedures described in (7) under Massage of the Chest (see page 88).

(14) Superficial Stroking.

Follow the procedures described in (1) (see pages 102–103).

HEAD

(1) Digital Kneading over the Head.

The thumbs are placed at the temples, the fingers are spread apart, and the finger tips are placed on either side of the medial line of the scalp to knead with firm pressure in small circles, in sections, until the entire head is covered. The finger tips keep contact with the skin and move the scalp over the bony surface. The pressure must be released before the finger tips are moved to each succeeding area, in order to avoid "pulling" the hair.

BACK OF NECK

*(1) Superficial and then Deep Stroking over the Upper
Fibers of the Trapezius (Bilateral).*

The thumbs are placed on the borders of the trapezius muscles, lateral to the spinous processes of the upper cervical vertebrae, and with the palms of the hands in contact over the tops of the shoulders. Both hands stroke lightly to the acromia, picking up the muscle as the thumbs reach the lower cervical region. The hands return to the starting position with a superficial stroke.

This movement is done eight times, with increasing pressure, so that by the fifth stroke the physical therapist is doing deep stroking, with the hands returning to the starting position with superficial stroking.

*(2) Digital Kneading over the Upper fibers
of the Trapezii.*

The finger tips of the right hand (which is reinforced with the left hand) are placed at the upper cervical region of the left trapezius. They knead in small clockwise circles, exerting heavier pressure when making the last half of each circle. Kneading progresses to the acromion process. The finger tips return to the starting position with a superficial stroke.
[Do this movement three times.]
The right side is kneaded in the same manner, except that the circles are made counterclockwise.
[Do this movement three times.]

*(3) Deep Stroking over the Upper Fibers of
the Trapezii.*

This movement is performed in the way described for (1) (see page 109), except that the pressure starts deep and is gradually lessened to superficial stroking.
[Do this movement six times.]

LOCAL MASSAGE

The use of massage in the local treatment of injury and other pathological changes in the muscles, tendons, joints, nerves, and blood vessels requires a thorough knowledge of the anatomy and physiology of these structures and an understanding of the pathology which exists in the tissues of the area to be treated.

The muscles may be atrophied, decreased in tone, fibrosed, flaccid, or in spasm;

edema may be present; the joints may be inflamed; motion may be limited by pain, adhesions, or contractures; the tendons may be adherent to the surrounding structures; the circulation may be impaired. Each of these conditions must be recognized and treated by a precise technique selected according to the changes that are present and the effects that are desired.

The technique of massage for this type of treatment requires the ability to recognize by palpation the condition of the tissues and to select and apply massage movements carefully and intelligently, adapting them to the condition in a purposeful manner. Mennell believed the physical therapist should be able to give a reason for each massage movement used.

Hoffa System

The Hoffa system of massage is well adapted to the treatment of many pathological conditions.

Hoffa was greatly interested in scientific massage and emphasized the importance of training physicians at universities and orthopedic clinics to appreciate its value. Hoffa's *Technic der Massage* was published in four editions, the last in 1903. The system that this eminent surgeon developed by his own use of massage follows an anatomical pattern and is based on a knowledge of physiology.

The movements are applied to certain muscles or muscle groups, as contrasted to movements applied either to an entire extremity or to a certain area of the body, as in some other systems. Hoffa classified the essential movements as effleurage (stroking), friction, pétrissage (kneading), vibration, and tapotement (percussion) and stated that these are only the framework on which an experienced physical therapist with good judgment may build up an effective treatment for the conditions present in any case. He emphasized the value of massage to increase the venous and lymphatic circulation.

According to Hoffa, effleurage (stroking) is employed to affect the circulation of the small veins in the muscles and particularly the large veins or venous plexuses which lie in the grooves between the individual muscles. This is accomplished by making the hand conform closely to the contour of the part, the thumb and finger tips simultaneously proceeding along these interstices.

Friction movements are applied chiefly to break down pathological exudates, deposits, and thickenings of tissue around the joints, tendons, and tendon sheaths and to assist in removing the waste products through the lymphatic system.

Pétrissage (kneading) is used chiefly to increase the circulation in the muscles and to remove "fatigue products" in a manner similar to friction.

Vibration and tapotement (Percussion) are recommended to increase blood supply, lessen nerve irritability, and increase contraction of muscle fiber. The author believes (see page 46) that these movements are of very little use in the treatment of such disease and injury.

Classification and Description of Local Massage Movements

The following classification and description of massage movements are the author's modifications of the Hoffa system of massage.

STROKING

(1) The direction of the deep stroke is always in the direction of the venous flow when an extremity is being massaged.
(2) The stroke is applied to the entire length of the muscle or muscle group, beginning at the insertion and continuing to the origin.
(3) The hand returns over the same area with light pressure (superficial stroking).
(4) The hand is made to conform to the shape of the muscle or muscle group, attempting to reach around and lift up the bulk of the muscle or muscle group.

The palmar surfaces of the entire hand, the distal phalanges of the fingers, or the distal phalanx of the thumb are used, according to the size of the muscle.
(5) The pressure is regulated according to the bulk of the muscles: light at the beginning of the deep stroke, increasing over the bulk of the muscles, and diminishing at the end of the stroke, finishing with a "squeeze-out" movement. In performing the "squeeze-out" movement, the grasping surfaces of the hand are gradually more closely approximated as the muscle bulk decreases and the hand approaches the origin of the muscle. As the hand reaches the point of origin, it is turned into the pronated position. The bulk of the tissue being massaged is thus "squeezed out" of the hand, and the hand is in position to start the return stroke.
(6) The movements should be performed rhythmically.
(7) The rate of movement should be that previously described under general massage (see pages 38, 42).

KNEADING

The kneading movements are performed with one or both hands (one-hand or two-hand kneading), or with the distal phalanx of the thumb, index, and middle fingers of one or both hands (digital kneading). One-hand kneading is used on muscles that are not too large to be grasped in one hand. For large massive muscles, two-hand kneading is used. Digital kneading is used on narrow or flat muscles that cannot be grasped easily by the entire hand. As in stroking, the hand must conform to the size and shape of the muscles and make firm contact. The movement begins at the insertion of the muscle and is carried through to the origin.

One-hand Kneading

(a) The hand is placed at the insertion of the muscle with the palmar surface of its ulnar border in firm contact (Fig. 151, page 113)
(b) The hand grasps around the bulk of the muscle and lifts it as much as possible from the underlying tissues (Fig. 152, page 113)
(c) The fingers and ulnar border of the hand follow along one border of the muscle or muscle group, and the thumb follows along the opposite border (Fig. 152, page 113)
(d) The movement is one of grasping and releasing the tissues and is carried through to the origin of the muscle, finishing with a "squeeze-out" movement (Fig. 161, page 116)
(e) The thumb and fingers work simultaneously but the pressure must be diminished as they approach each other, to prevent pinching.
(f) Care must be used to keep the bulk of the muscle well back in the palm of the hand between the thenar eminence and the metacarpal pad of the palm (Fig. 152, page 113).
(g) At the origin of the muscle, the hand is brought over into pronation and returned to the starting position with a superficial stroke over the area (Fig. 201 and 202, page 128)

Two-hand Kneading

(a) One hand is placed at the insertion of the muscle as in one-hand kneading; the other hand is placed just proximal to it (Fig. 199, page 128)
(b) Both hands grasp around as much of the muscle as possible. The palmar surface of the fingers of the left hand pulls the muscles laterally as the surface of the abducted right thumb and palm simultaneously pushes the tissues medially. Then the surface of the palm and abducted thumb of the left hand pushes the muscles medially as the palmar surface of the fingers of the right hand pulls the tissues laterally (Fig. 153, page 114). Progression from the distal to the proximal part of the muscle is accomplished with a gliding of the hands on the "pull" stroke of the kneading movement.

This is not a pinching type of movement. The thumb and fingers of each hand are kept in the same relationship to each other during the entire movement. The "push" and "pull" are accomplished chiefly by flexion and extension of the arms at the shoulders and elbows. At the origin, the proximal hand is removed, and the distal hand finishes with the "squeeze-out" movement (Figs. 201 and 202, page 128) and returns to starting position with a superficial stroke, as in one-hand kneading.

Two-hand Digital Kneading

The muscle is grasped at its insertion by both hands (between the thumb and index and middle fingers of each hand). The palmar surface of the left fingers pulls the tissues toward the physical therapist while the right thumb pushes the adjacent tissues away. Then the right fingers pull the tissues while the left thumb pushes the adjacent tissues (Fig. 211, page 131). Progression from origin to insertion is accomplished with a gliding of the fingers on the "pull" movement.

This is not a pinching movement. The thumb and fingers of each hand are kept in the same relationship to each other during the entire movement. The "push" and "pull" are accomplished chiefly by flexion and extension of the arms at the shoulders and elbows. The return stroke is performed with the fingers of the distal hand.

This movement is used on muscles of small bulk. Care must be taken that the hands are held as nearly parallel to the length of the muscles as is possible and with as much contact as is possible.

FRICTION

The description of friction and the indications for its use have been considered elsewhere (see page 45 and 46). It is applicable in local massage for the treatment of scars and adhesions of tendons and joints.

Technique for Local Massage

The technique of local massage that follows and its application to the anatomical sections of the body are the author's modifications of the Hoffa system.

In the application of the massage movements to the anatomical sections of an extremity, the proximal portion should be treated first and then the more distal segment or segments (see page 65). Following this, special attention may be given to areas requiring additional treatment. The stroking and kneading movements may be adapted to conform to the muscles of any area of the body. In the beginning of treatment, stroking precedes the kneading movement, and periods of stroking and kneading (or stroking and friction) should alternate according to the pathological condition in the tissues, the effect desired, and the result being obtained from the massage. The final movement should always be stroking.

The order in which the massage is given to the various muscle groups of each anatomical section will depend upon the condition being treated and upon the ability of the patient to be moved into the required positions. It may be necessary to alter the techniques of the movements slightly in order to avoid unnecessary changes of the patient's position, as, for instance, in the treatment of fractures. In general, the position of the patient should be changed as little as possible. The techniques, as described, are those that should be followed when it is possible to place the patient in the ideal position to perform the movements.

The patient should under most circumstances be recumbent while receiving massage treatment (see page 63).

RIGHT ARM

The therapist stands at the side of the table at the patient's right. The patient is supine, with the right upper extremity slightly abducted.

The arm is divided into three muscle groups: deltoid, extensor, and flexor.

(1) Deltoid Muscle Group.

Stroking: The hands stroke alternately. Beginning at the insertion of the muscle (Fig. 147), the thumb of each hand passes up the midline of the muscle; the fingers of the left hand follow the posterior border of the muscle and curve around the origin to the center (Fig. 148); the fingers of the right hand follow the anterior border in the same manner (Fig. 149). Each hand returns to its starting position with a superficial stroke (Fig. 150).

If the muscle is small, the entire muscle may be stroked with the left hand, as the right hand supports the inner side of the upper arm. The fingers of the left hand follow the posterior border of the muscle, and the thumb follows the anterior border of the muscle (Fig. 151); they meet at the acromion in a "squeeze-out" movement (Fig. 152). The left hand returns to its starting position with a superficial stroke.

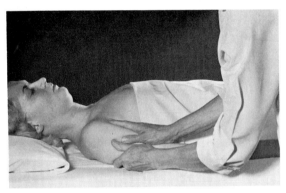

Figure 147

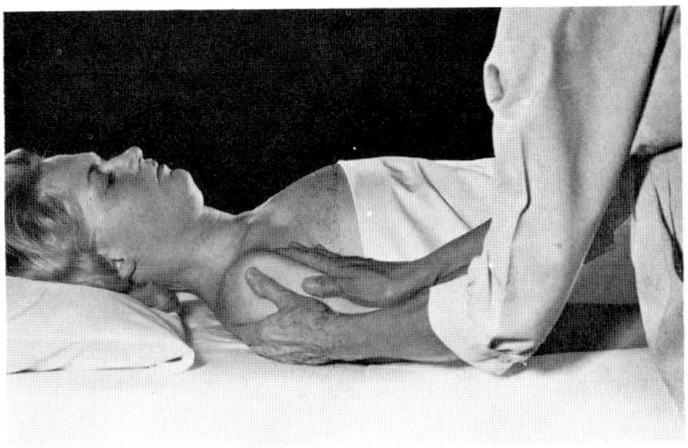

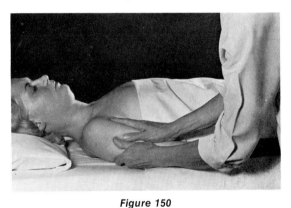

Figure 148

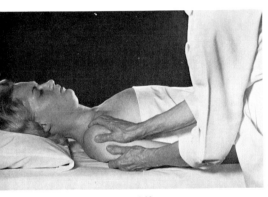

Figure 149

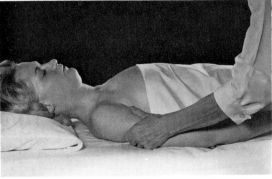

Figure 150

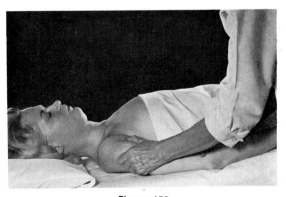

Figure 151

Figure 152

(1) Deltoid Muscle Group—Continued

Kneading: Two-hand kneading is done to the entire muscle, with the patient's arm in partial abduction. Kneading progresses from the insertion to the origin of the muscle (Fig. 153). The left hand does a "squeeze-out" movement at the origin and returns to the starting position with a superficial stroke, as the right hand returns through the air.

One-hand kneading may be done with the left hand if the muscle is small; the right hand gives support to the arm (Fig. 154).

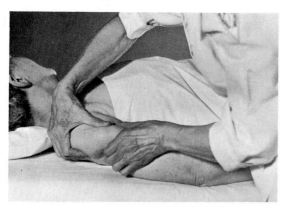

Figure 153

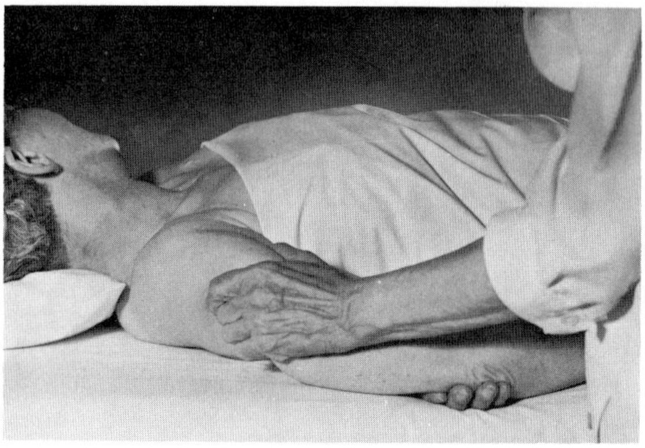

Figure 154

(2) Extensor Muscle Group (Triceps and Anconeus).

Stroking: The right hand supports the elbow; the left hand grasps around the muscle group at the insertion. The thumb follows the lateral border and the fingers the medial border of the triceps as the hand strokes over the muscle (Fig. 155). At the end of the stroke, the thumb passes around the posterior border of the deltoid while the fingers move into the axilla, as the hand does a "squeeze-out" movement (Fig. 156). The hand then returns to the starting position with a superficial stroke.

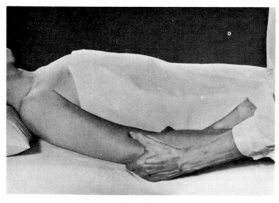

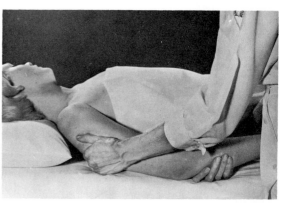

Figure 155

Figure 156

*(2) Extensor Muscle Group (Triceps and
Anconeus)—Continued.*

Kneading: One-hand kneading is done over the same area as the stroking (Figs. 157, 158), and the hand returns with a superficial stroke.

Two-hand kneading may be used if the muscle group is large. The patient's arm is partially abducted and both hands grasp the triceps, the left hand at the insertion and the right hand just proximal to it (Fig. 159).

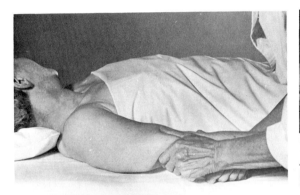
Figure 157

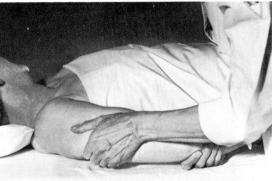
Figure 158

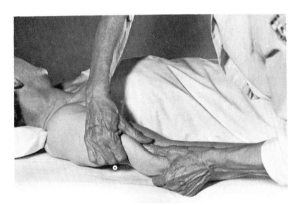
Figure 159

(3) Flexor Muscle Group (Biceps, Brachialis, and Coracobrachialis).

Stroking: The left hand supports the elbow, and the right hand grasps the muscle group at its insertion below the elbow joint (Fig. 160). The thumb follows the lateral border and the fingers the medial border of the flexor muscle group, as the hand strokes over the muscles. At the end of the stroke, the thumb passes around the anterior border of the deltoid, while the fingers move into the axilla as the hand does a "squeeze-out" movement (Fig. 161). The hand then returns to the starting position with a superficial stroke.

Kneading: One-hand kneading is done over the same area as the stroking (Fig. 162). Two-hand kneading may be used if the muscle group is large. Hand positions are the reverse of those described for two-hand kneading of the triceps group (Fig. 159).

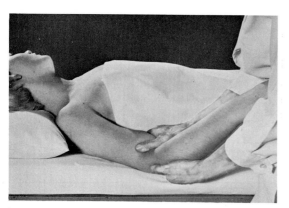

Figure 160

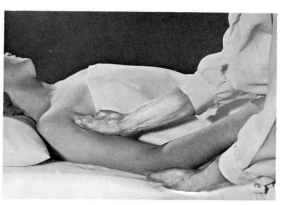

Figure 161

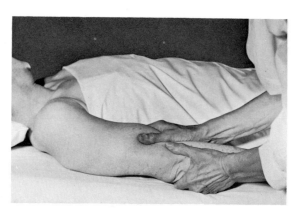

Figure 162

RIGHT FOREARM

The forearm is divided into two muscle groups; medial and lateral.

(1) Medial Muscle Group.

The patient's elbow is slightly flexed, with the forearm in supination while the arm rests on the table.

Stroking: The left hand supports the forearm at the wrist. The right hand starts the stroke by grasping around the medial half of the forearm at the wrist (Fig. 163). The thumb then passes up the midline of the forearm to the elbow and over the medial condyle as the fingers pass up along the ulna and over the medial condyle to meet the thumb in a "squeeze-out" movement (Fig. 164). The hand returns to the wrist with a superficial stroke.

Kneading: One-hand kneading is done over the same area as the stroking (Figs. 165, 166), and the hand returns with a superficial stroke.

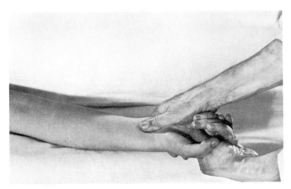

Figure 163

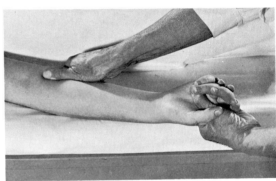

Figure 164

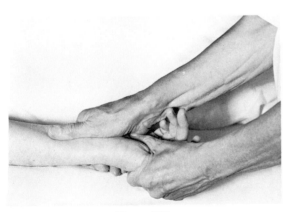

Figure 165

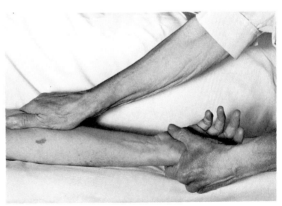

Figure 166

(2) Lateral Muscle Group.

Stroking: The right hand supports the wrist. The left hand starts the stroke by grasping around the lateral half of the forearm (Fig. 167). The thumb then passes up the midline of the forearm to the elbow and over the lateral condyle as the fingers pass along the radius and over the lateral condyle to meet the thumb in a "squeeze-out" movement (Fig. 168). The hand returns to the wrist with a superficial stroke.

Kneading: One-hand kneading is done over the same area as the stroking (Figs. 169, 170), and the hand returns with a superficial stroke.

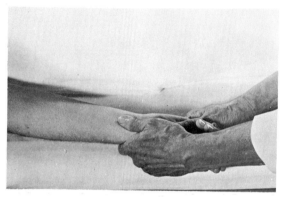

Figure 167

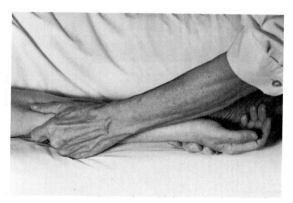

Figure 168

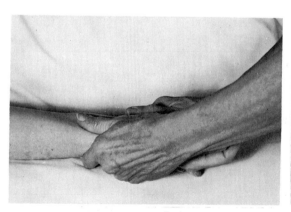

Figure 169

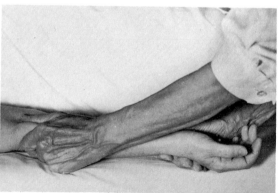

Figure 170

RIGHT HAND

(1) Muscles of the Radial Border.

The patient's forearm and hand are in supination, with the thumb abducted and the forearm supported on the table.

Stroking: The therapist's right hand supports the patient's hand. The left hand grasps the radial half of the hand at the metacarpophalangeal joint. The thumb then passes up the midline of the palm (Fig. 171) around the thenar eminence to the wrist. The fingers pass up the midline of the dorsal surface of the hand to join the thumb at the wrist with a "squeeze-out" movement. The hand returns with a superficial stroke.

Kneading: One-hand kneading is done over the same area as the stroking (Fig. 171), and the hand returns with a superficial stroke.

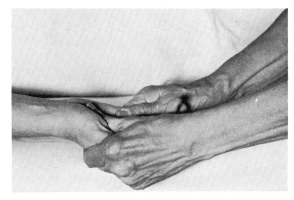

Figure 171

2) Muscles of the Ulnar Border.

Stroking: The therapist's left hand supports the patient's hand. The right hand grasps the ulnar half of the patient's hand at the metacarpophalangeal joint. The thumb then passes up the midline of the palm (Fig. 172) around the hypothenar eminence to the wrist. The fingers pass up the midline of the dorsal surface of the hand to meet the thumb at the wrist with a "squeeze-out" movement. The hand returns with a superficial stroke.

Kneading: One-hand kneading is done over the same area as the stroking (Fig. 173), and the hand returns with a superficial stroke.

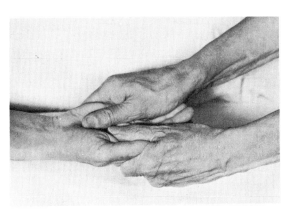

Figure 172

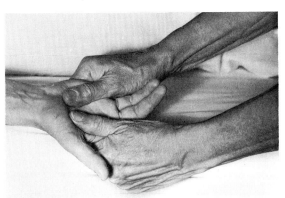

Figure 173

(3) Volar Surface.

The patient's hand is in supination.

Stroking: The patient's hand is supported by the therapist's right hand while the thumb of the left hand strokes over each of the following areas: the thenar eminence from the first metacarpophalangeal joint to the wrist (Fig. 174); the interossei and the lumbricales from the metacarpophalangeal joints to the wrist (Fig. 175); and the hypothenar eminence, from the fifth metacarpophalangeal joint to the wrist (Fig. 176). The thumb returns with a superficial stroke after each movement.

Kneading: The thumb kneads in small circles over the same areas and in the same order as indicated in the stroking (Figs. 174, 175, 176) and returns with a superficial stroke.

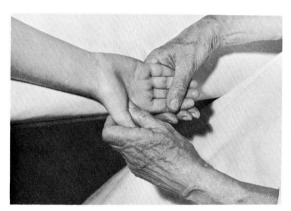

Figure 174

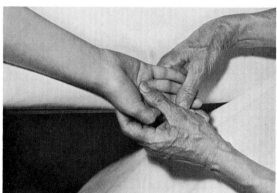

Figure 175

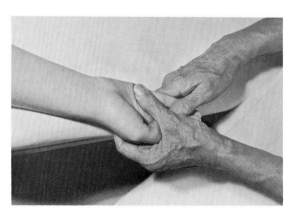

Figure 176

(4) Dorsal Surface.

The patient's hand is in pronation.

Stroking: The patient's hand is supported by the therapist's left hand. The thumb of the right hand strokes over the ulnar side of the first metacarpal, just proximal to the first interphalangeal joint and continuing to the wrist (Fig. 177). It returns with a superficial stroke along the radial side of the second metacarpal to its first interphalangeal joint; it strokes over this same area to the wrist. The thumb then slides over so that it can return along the ulnar border of the second metacarpal to the first interphalangeal joint and then strokes over the same area to the wrist.

The same procedures are done for the third and fourth metacarpal areas, and the radial side of the fifth metacarpal. Obviously, the thumb will be stroking in the interosseus spaces between the metacarpals, with pressure directed to the interosseus muscles.

Kneading: The thumb kneads in small circles over each interosseous muscle from the insertion to the wrist, following the routine described for stroking.

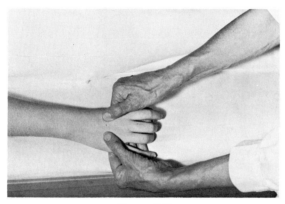

Figure 177

RIGHT THUMB AND FINGERS

(1) Dorsal Surface.

The patient's hand is in pronation.

The patient's hand is supported on the volar surface by the fingers of the left hand (Fig. 178). These fingers also support the phalanges as needed to prevent flexion during these movements. The right thumb and index finger first stroke, then knead the thumb and each succeeding finger as follows:

Thumb stroking: The thumb and the index finger grasp around the tip (Fig. 178) of the patient's digit, the index finger passes up the radial side of the digit to the metacarpophalangeal joint as the thumb passes up the ulnar side (Figs. 179, 180) and continues the stroke into the metacarpal-interosseus space (Fig. 181). The thumb and the finger return to the tip of the digit with a superficial stroke.

Thumb kneading: The finger supports, while the thumb kneads over the same area as it stroked (Figs. 182, 183). They return to the tip of the digit with a superficial stroke. The therapist's hand is then supinated so that the thumb can knead on the radial side of the patient's digit, while the index finger supports on the ulnar side (Fig. 184). The thumb and the finger return to the tip of the digit with a superficial stroke.

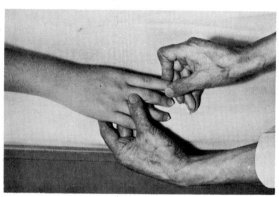

Figure 178

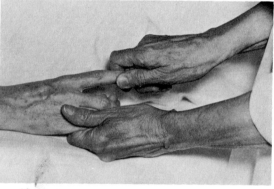

Figure 179

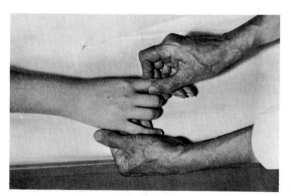

Figure 180

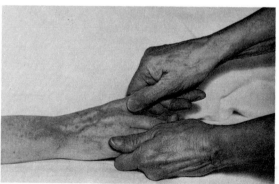

Figure 181

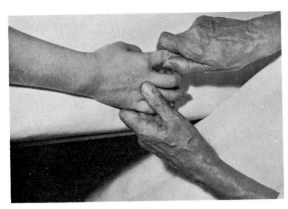

Figure 182

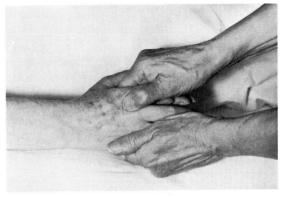

Figure 183

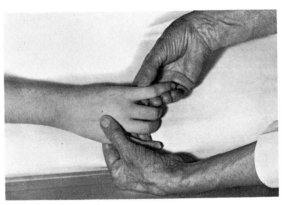

Figure 184

(2) Volar Surface.

The patient's hand is in supination.

Stroking and kneading: The patient's hand is supported on the dorsal surface by the fingers of the left hand (Fig. 185). The right thumb and the index finger first stroke (Figs. 185, 186) and then knead (Figs. 187, 188) the thumb and the fingers in the same manner as was done on the dorsal surface, except that they start with the little finger and work to the thumb.

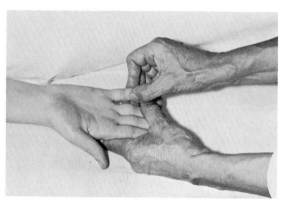

Figure 185

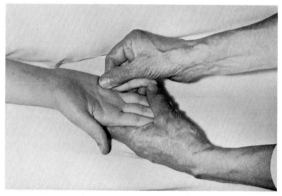

Figure 186

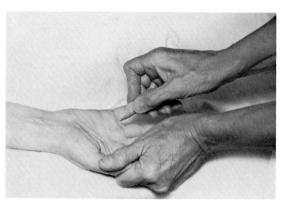

Figure 187

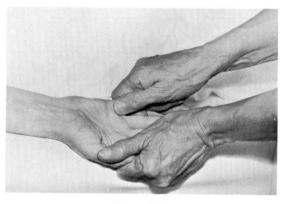

Figure 188

LEFT UPPER EXTREMITY

The therapist stands at the side of the table on the patient's left. The movements are performed as described for the right upper extremity, except that the right hand is substituted for the left, and the left hand for the right.

RIGHT BUTTOCKS

The therapist stands at the side of the table on the patient's right. The patient is prone, with a pillow under the abdomen and one under the ankles; the head may be turned to either side for comfort.

(1) Gluteal Muscle Group.

Stroking: The left hand starts the stroke at the insertion of the gluteus maximus into the fascia lata (Fig. 189) and follows the fibers of this muscle to its origin at the sacrum, coccyx, and ilium (along the gluteal fold). The right hand follows the fibers of the gluteus medius from its insertion at the greater trochanter to its origin on the crest of the ilium (Fig. 189). The hands stroke alternately and return with a superficial stroke.

If the muscles are large, each muscle may be stroked separately. In this instance, the thumbs of the hands pass up the midline of the muscle being stroked.

*Kneading:*Two-hand kneading is done over the same area as the stroking (Fig. 190). At the end of the stroke, the right hand does a "squeeze-out" movement and returns with a superficial stroke, as the left hand returns through the air.

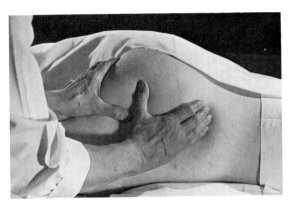

Figure 189

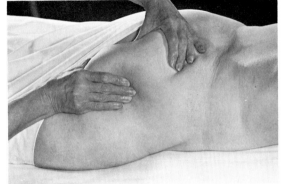

Figure 190

RIGHT THIGH

The therapist stands at the side of the table on the patient's right. The patient is prone.

(1) Inner Hamstring Group
(Semimembranosus and Semitendinosus).

Stroking: The right hand supports the extremity (Fig. 191). The left hand begins at the insertion of the muscles just below the medial condyle of the tibia and grasps around the muscle group (Fig. 191). The thumb follows up the midline of the thigh as the fingers follow the medial border of the muscle group to meet the thumb at the gluteal fold in a "squeeze-out" movement (Fig. 192). The hand returns with a superficial stroke.

Kneading: Two-hand kneading is done over the same area as the stroking.

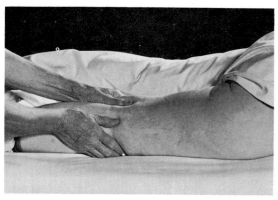
Figure 191

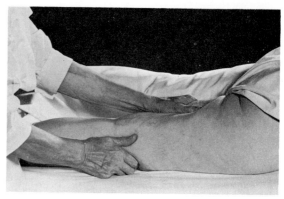
Figure 192

(2) Outer Hamstring Group (Biceps Femoris).

Stroking: The left hand supports the extremity. The right hand begins at the insertion of the muscle on the head of the fibula and grasps around the muscle (Fig. 193). The thumb passes up the midline of the thigh; the fingers follow the lateral border of the muscle to meet the thumb at the gluteal fold in a "squeeze-out" movement (Fig. 194). The hand returns with a superficial stroke.

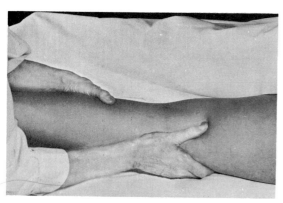
Figure 193

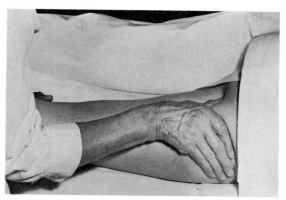
Figure 194

Kneading: Two-hand kneading is done over the same area as the stroking. One-hand kneading may be used for both inner and outer hamstring groups if the muscles are small.

Note: The stroking and kneading movements to both inner and outer hamstring muscles may also be done with the patient supine or lying on his side, if it is not advisable to have the patient turn to the prone position. In the supine position, one hand supports the knee in slight flexion while the other hand performs the movement.

(3) Tensor Fasciae Latae.

The therapist stands at the side of the table on the patient's right. The patient is supine.

Stroking: The right hand gives support to the thigh at the medial side of the knee (Fig. 195). The left hand starts the stroke at the insertion of the fasciae latae on the head of the fibula (Fig. 195). The thumb follows the anterior border of the fascia and muscle, and the fingers follow the posterior border of the fascia and muscle, as the hand strokes toward the origin. As the hand approaches the muscular portion, it spreads out to stroke over the muscle to its origin (Fig. 196), and finishes with a "squeeze-out" movement. The hand returns with a superficial stroke.

Kneading: Two-hand kneading is done over the same area as the stroking. One-hand kneading may be done if the muscle is small.

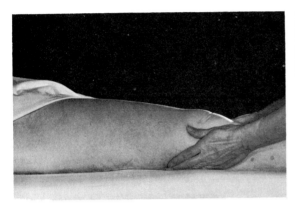

Figure 195

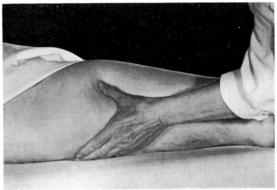

Figure 196

(4) Quadriceps Muscle Group.

Stroking: The right hand supports the extremity at the knee. The left hand is placed below the patella at the insertion of the muscle, with the thumb at the medial border and the fingers at the lateral border of the patella (Fig. 197). The hand passes lightly over the patella, grasps around the muscle, and strokes to its origin, where the thumb and fingers meet in a "squeeze-out" movement (Fig. 198). The hand returns with a superficial stroke.

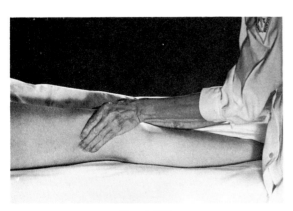

Figure 197

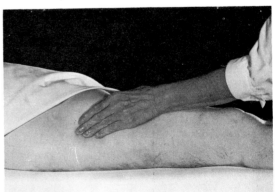

Figure 198

(4) Quadriceps Muscle Group—Continued.

*Kneading:*The right hand is placed at the lower border of the patella and passes lightly over the patella; the left hand picks up the muscle above the patella (Fig. 199), and both hands knead the entire muscle to its origin (Fig. 200). The right hand performs a "squeeze-out" movement (Fig. 201) and returns with a superficial stroke (Fig. 202). The left hand returns through the air.

One-hand kneading may be done if the muscle group is small (Figs. 203, 204). Kneading is done with the left hand, and the right hand gives support to the extremity.

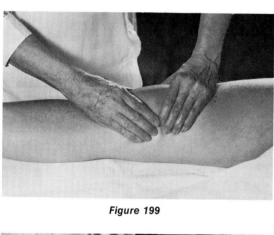

Figure 199

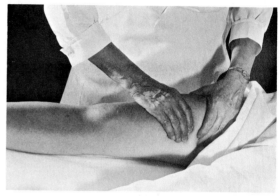

Figure 200

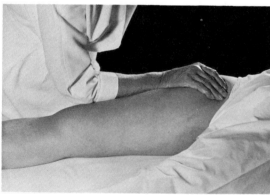

Figure 201

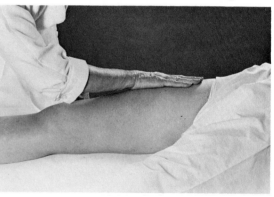

Figure 202

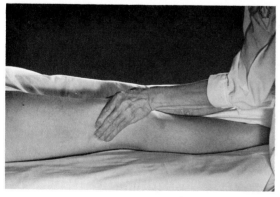

Figure 203

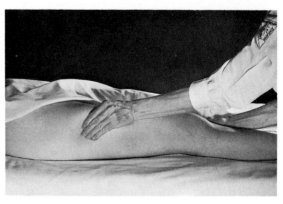

Figure 204

(5) Adductor Muscle Group.

Stroking: The right hand, reinforced by the left hand, starts the stroke at the insertion of the muscle group on the medial condyle of the tibia and grasps around the muscle group (Fig. 205). The thumb passes up the anterior border of the muscle group and the fingers follow the posterior border toward the origin, finishing with a "squeeze-out" movement. Theoretically this should end at the origin of the muscle, but practically it should be completed about two inches distal to the origin because of the cremaster reflex (Fig. 206). The hand returns with a superficial stroke.

Kneading: Two-hand kneading is done over the same area as the stroking. The right hand does a "squeeze-out" movement at the end of the kneading and returns with a superficial stroke. The left hand returns through the air.

One-hand kneading may be used on a small muscle. If so, the left hand reinforces the right hand.

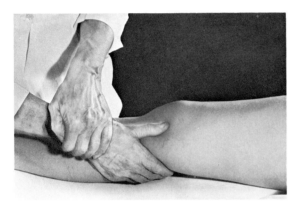

Figure 205

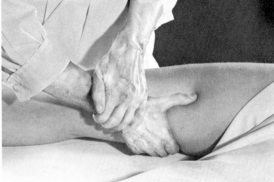

Figure 206

RIGHT LEG

The therapist stands at the foot of the table.

(1) Anterior Muscle Group.

Stroking: The left hand is placed slightly distal to the ankle joint and the right hand supports the ankle by grasping the foot at the arch. The left thumb passes along the lateral border of the tibia, and the index finger follows the lateral border of the muscle group (Fig. 207) to the anterior surface of the head of the fibula to meet the thumb in a "squeeze-out" movement. (The other fingers maintain light contact with the skin throughout the movement.) The hand returns to the starting position with a superficial stroke.

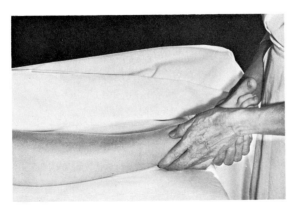

Figure 207

(1) Anterior Muscle Group—Continued.

Kneading: Two-hand digital kneading is done over the same area as the stroking. The therapist may stay at the foot of the table and turn his body so that the hands reach across the tibia to knead the muscles. The right hand is placed proximally and the left hand distally (Fig. 208). The left hand does the "squeeze out" at the end of the movement and returns with a superficial stroke while the right hand returns in the air.

Or the therapist may move to the right side of the table and do two-hand kneading, with the left hand placed proximally and the right hand distally. The right hand does the "squeeze out" at the end of the movement and returns with a superficial stroke, while the left hand returns in the air.

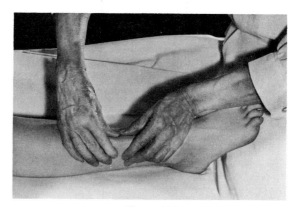

Figure 208

(2) Peroneal Muscle Group.

Stroking: The left hand is placed distal to the lateral malleolus and the right hand supports the ankle by grasping the foot at the arch (Fig. 209). The left thumb follows the anterior border of the muscle group and the index finger follows along the posterior border of the muscle group (Fig. 210) to the posterior surface of the head of the fibula to meet the thumb in a "squeeze-out" movement. The hand returns to the starting position with a superficial stroke. (The other fingers maintain light contact with the skin throughout the movement.)

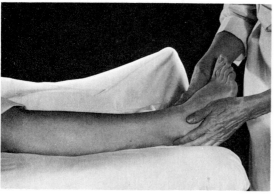
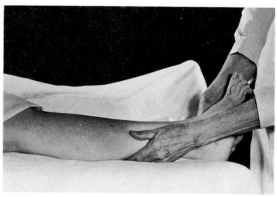

Figure 209   **Figure 210**

(2) Peroneal Muscle Group—Continued.

*Kneading:*Two-hand digital kneading is done over the same area as the stroking. Procedures are similar to those described for two-hand digital kneading of the anterior muscle group (Fig. 211).

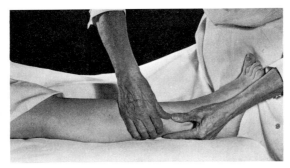

Figure 211

(3) Posterior Muscle Group.

The therapist stands at the side of the table on the patient's right. The patient is prone.

*Stroking:*The left hand is placed on the heel and the right hand stabilizes the leg at the knee (Fig. 212). The left thumb follows along the lateral border of the tendo achillis and passes up the lateral border of the muscle group as the fingers follow along the medial border of the tendon and muscle group. The hand grasps around the muscle group and strokes toward the origins of the gastrocnemius. The first stroke ends in a "squeeze-out" movement over the medial head (Fig. 213); the second stroke ends in a "squeeze-out" movement over the lateral head (Fig. 214). Additional strokes continue to alternate at the finish. The hand returns to the starting position with a superficial stroke.

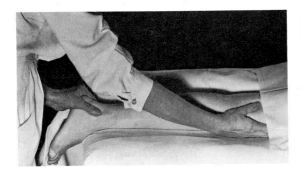

Figure 212

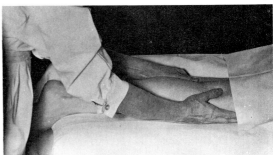

Figure 213

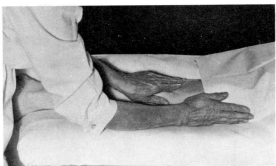

Figure 214

(3) Posterior Muscle Group—Continued.

If the muscle group is too large to be grasped in one hand, it may be massaged in two sections. The medial side of the muscle group is stroked with the left hand, as the right hand supports the knee (Fig. 215). The left thumb passes up the midline of the muscle group, and the "squeeze out" is done at the medial head of the gastrocnemius. The lateral side of the muscle group is stroked with the right hand, as the left hand supports the knee (Fig. 216). The "squeeze out" is done at the lateral head of the gastrocnemius.

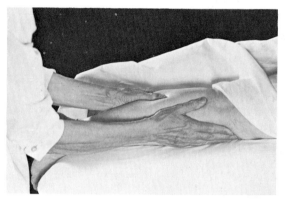

Figure 215

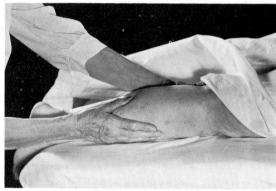

Figure 216

Kneading: Two-hand kneading is done to the same area as the stroking (Fig. 217). The left hand returns to the starting position with a superficial stroke, and the right hand returns in the air.

If the muscle group is very large, two-hand kneading is done over each half of the muscle group (Fig. 218).

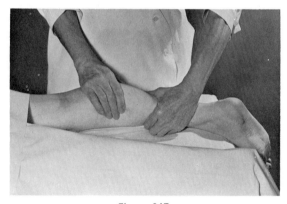

Figure 217

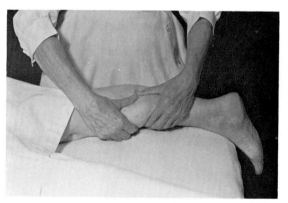

Figure 218

If the muscle group is small, one-hand kneading may be used over the whole muscle group. The left hand kneads as the right hand supports the extremity.

(3) Posterior Muscle Group—Continued.

If it is not advisable to have the patient in the prone position, this muscle group may be massaged with the patient supine. With the patient in this position, one hand supports the knee in slight flexion while the other does the stroking movement (Fig. 219).

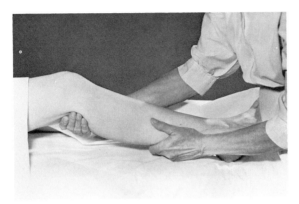

Figure 219

Two-hand kneading is done with the therapist standing at the side of the table on the patient's right. The patient's thigh is laterally rotated, so that both hands can grasp the muscle group easily (Fig. 220). If the muscle group is small, one-hand kneading may be done with the left hand, as the right hand supports the knee in slight flexion (Fig. 221).

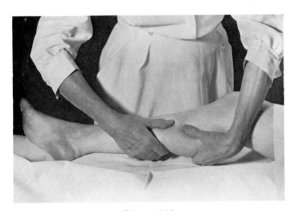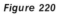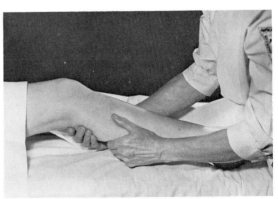

Figure 220   *Figure 221*

RIGHT FOOT

The therapist stands at the foot of the table. The patient is supine.

(1) Medial Border.

Stroking: The left hand supports the ankle on the lateral side, just proximal to the heel (Fig. 222). The right hand grasps the medial half of the foot at the toes. The thumb passes up the midline of the dorsum of the foot and below the medial malleolus, as the fingers pass up the midline of the plantar surface and around the heel to meet the thumb in a "squeeze-out" movement (Fig. 223). The hand returns to the starting position with a superficial stroke.

Kneading: One-hand kneading is done over the same area as the stroking. The hand returns to the starting position with a superficial stroke.

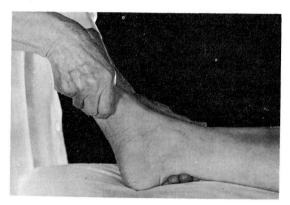

Figure 222   Figure 223

(2) Lateral Border.

Stroking: The right hand supports the ankle on the medial side, just proximal to the heel. The left hand grasps the lateral half of the foot at the toes (Fig. 224). The thumb passes up the midline of the dorsum of the foot and below the lateral malleolus, as the fingers pass up the midline of the plantar surface and around the heel to meet the thumb in a "squeeze-out" movement (Fig. 225). The hand returns to the starting position with a superficial stroke.

Kneading: One-hand kneading is done over the same area as the stroking. The hand returns to the starting position with a superficial stroke.

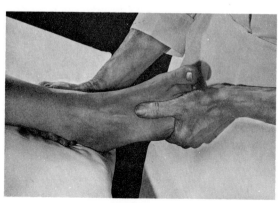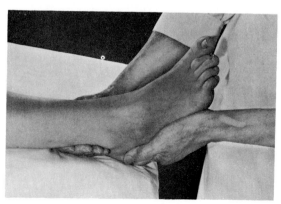

Figure 224   Figure 225

(3) Dorsal Surface.

Stroking: The fingers of both hands are placed on the plantar surface of the foot to support it. The thumbs perform short alternate strokes between the first and second metatarsal bones, progressing from the base of the toes to the ankle (Figs. 226, 227). Both thumbs together return to the starting position with a superficial stroke. They repeat the movements in each metatarsal space.

Kneading: Kneading is done with one thumb in small circles over the same area as the stroking. (The right thumb kneads over the first and second metatarsal spaces and the left thumb kneads over the third and fourth metatarsal spaces.) The thumb returns to the starting position with a superficial stroke.

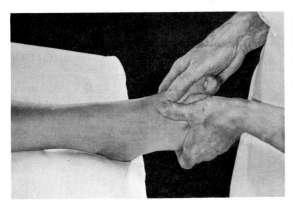

Figure 226

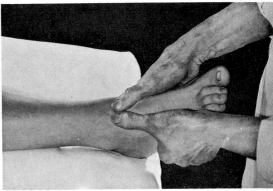

Figure 227

(4) Plantar Surface.

Stroking: The left hand supports the foot by grasping the forefoot and toes so that the dorsal surface of the foot fits into the palm of the left hand (Fig. 228). The fingers of the right hand are flexed at the metacarpophalangeal and the proximal phalangeal joints; the proximal phalanges are placed in firm contact at the base of the toes (Fig. 228). The hand strokes *firmly* toward the heel (Fig. 229). As the movement progresses, the right hand is rolled into pronation (Fig. 230) and the fingers are extended to allow the heel of the hand to fit into the longitudinal arch of the foot. The right hand is removed and returned through the air to the starting position.

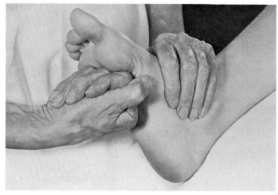
Figure 228

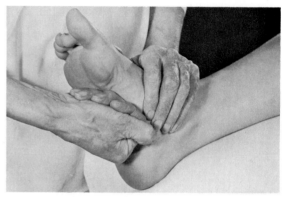
Figure 229

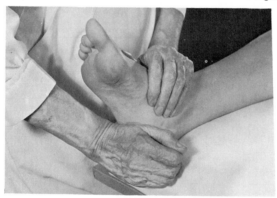
Figure 230

RIGHT TOES

If there is reason to massage the toes, stroking and kneading procedures similar to those described for the thumb and fingers (see pages 122–124) are used.

Note: If the therapist is asked to massage the lower extremity after a cast has been bi-valved for treatment of the extremity, all of the movements that can be done in the prone position should follow one another. Then (after the patient has been properly turned) all of the movements that can be done in the supine position should follow.

LEFT LOWER EXTREMITY

The therapist stands at the patient's left side. The movements are done as described for the right lower extremity, except that the right hand is substituted for the left and the left hand is substituted for the right.

BACK

The therapist stands at the side of the table on the patient's left side. The patient is prone.

Local massage to the back is done to three muscle groups: erector spinae, trapezius and scapular, and latissimus dorsi. With the exception of stroking to the erector spinae group, all movements are done to one side of the back at a time.

(1) Erector Spinae Muscle Group.

Stroking: The thumbs are placed at the sides of the spinous processes of the up-per cervical vertebrae, and the fingers are placed in the supraclavicular fossae (Fig. 231). Both thumbs stroke down firmly over the cervical region and at the seventh cervical vertebra are lifted and crossed to give reinforcement to the hands (Fig. 232). The fingers are then lightly drawn backward toward the seventh cervical vertebra and the palms stroke firmly over the erector spinae muslces from the seventh cervical vertebra to the sacrum.

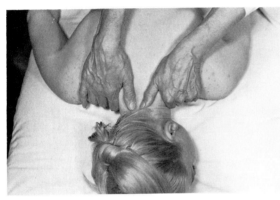

Figure 231

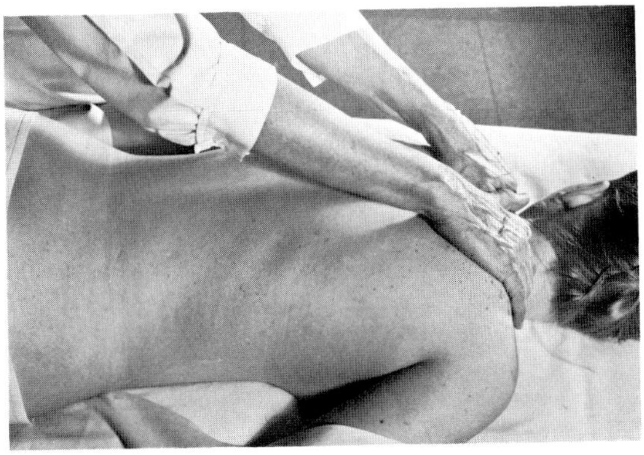

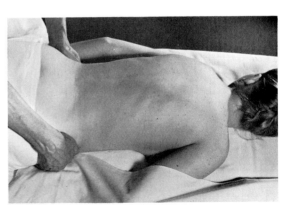

Figure 232

The hands then separate, and with thumbs adducted stroke with light pressure over the ilii (Fig. 233) to the inguinal region and return to the sacrum (Fig. 234). The hands then stroke back over the erector spinae muscles to the seventh cervical vertebra, the thumbs again being lifted and crossed. Light pressure is used for this return stroke.

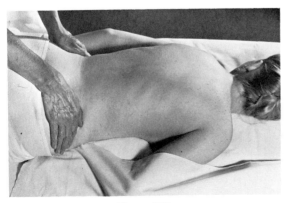

Figure 233

Figure 234

(1) Erector Spinae Muscle Group—Continued.

Kneading: Two-hand digital kneading is done first to the right side and then to the left side, beginning at the cervical region and continuing to the sacrum (Fig. 235). The right hand returns with a superficial stroke, as the left hand returns through the air.

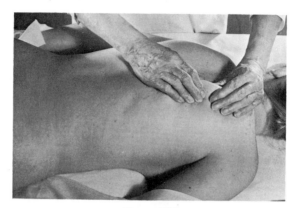

Figure 235

(2) Trapezius and Scapular Muscle Group.

Stroking: Starting on the right side, the right hand is placed over the upper fibers of the trapezius with the thumb at the lateral border of the upper cervical spinous processes; it grasps around the upper fibers of the right trapezius muscle and strokes to the acromion. As the right hand completes the stroke, the left hand is placed with the thumb abducted and its ulnar border beside the spinous processes (Fig. 236), and it strokes over the middle fibers of the trapezius to the acromion. Then the right hand, with the thumb abducted, is placed with the thumb beside the spinous processes and the ulnar border at the border of the lower trapezius fibers (at the level of the twelfth dorsal vertebra); it strokes from that position to the acromion. As it reaches the acromion, the left hand starts the first stroking movement, over the upper fibers of the trapezius. The right hand then strokes over the middle fibers (Fig. 237), then the left hand strokes over the lower fibers.

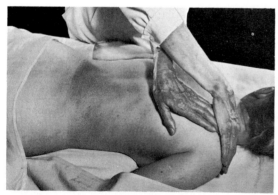

Figure 236

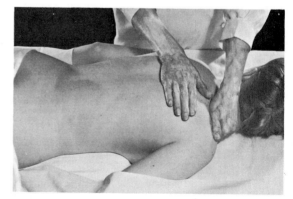

Figure 237

The movements are done in the same manner on the left side, except that the left hand substitutes for the right, and the right hand substitutes for the left.

(2) Trapezius and Scapular Muscle Group—Continued.

Kneading: Start on the right side.
(a) *Upper fibers.* Two-hand digital kneading is done over the same area as the stroking. The right hand returns with a superficial stroke, as the left hand returns through the air.
(b) *Middle and lower fibers.* Two-hand kneading is done over both areas (Fig. 238). The right hand returns with a superficial stroke, as the left hand returns through the air.

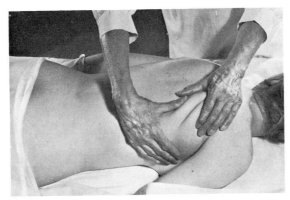

Figure 238

The movements are done in the same manner on the left side, except that the left hand substitutes for the right, and the right hand substitutes for the left.

(3) Latissimus Dorsi.

Stroking: Start on the right side. Place the right hand (reinforced by the left hand) with the thumb at the lateral border of the spinous processes of the lumbar area, and ulnar border on the crest of the ilium (Fig. 239). The thumb follows along the medial border of the muscle while the fingers follow along the lateral border. The hand turns into pronation as the fingers meet the thumb in the axilla in a "squeeze-out" movement (Fig. 240). The hand returns with a superficial stroke.

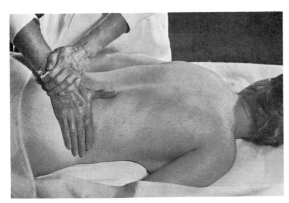

Figure 239

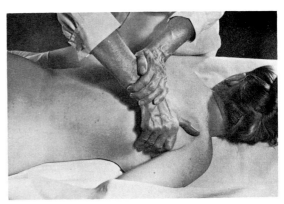

Figure 240

(3) Latissimus Dorsi—Continued.

Kneading: Two-hand kneading is done over the same area as the stroking (Fig. 241). The right hand returns with a superficial stroke as the left hand returns through the air.

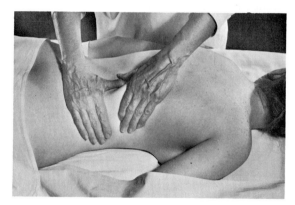

Figure 241

If the muscle is too large to be covered with one hand, the stroking and kneading may be done in two sections.

The movements are done in the same manner on the left side, except that the left hand substitutes for the right, and the right hand substitutes for the left.

ABDOMEN

The therapist stands at the side of the table on the patient's right. The patient is supine, with knees flexed and supported by pillows.

(1) Stroking over the Entire Abdomen.

Starting with the finger tips of both hands placed at the symphysis pubis (Fig. 242), the hands stroke over the rectus abdominus muscle to its origin (Fig. 243), then stroke laterally with light pressure (Fig. 244), fingers passing over the lower ribs. As the hands continue the lateral stroking over the dorsal part of the fibers, they turn (Fig. 245) so that the finger tips meet at the spine.

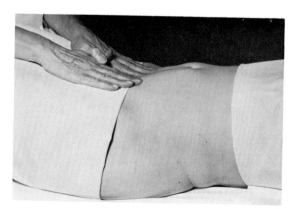

Figure 242

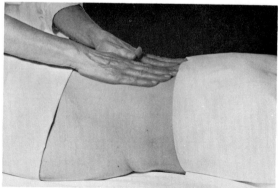

Figure 243

(1) Stroking over the Entire Abdomen — Continued.

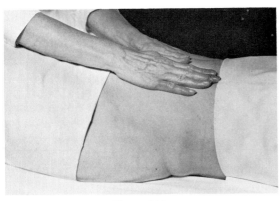

Figure 244

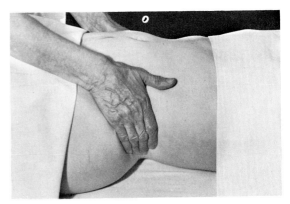

Figure 245

The hands then return over the same area with a firm stroke to the transverse abdominal muscles (Fig. 246), and a light stroke down the rectus abdominus to the symphysis pubis.

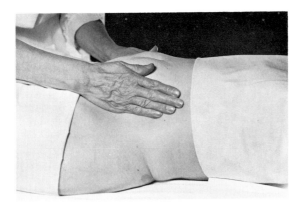

Figure 246

The stroking to the rectus abdominus and the lateral stroking are repeated, but the return stroke is over the oblique abdominal muscles (Fig. 247), toward the symphysis pubis.

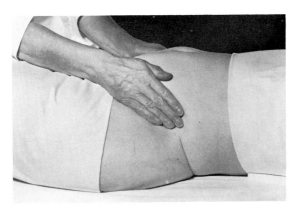

Figure 247

(2) Stroking over the Area of the Colon.

The finger tips of the right hand, reinforced with the left hand, are placed over the area of the cecum (Fig. 248). They stroke upward with firm pressure over the area of the ascending colon, across the abdomen over the area of the transverse colon, and downward over the area of the descending colon (Fig. 249). The hands return with a superficial stroke across the lower abdomen to the starting point.

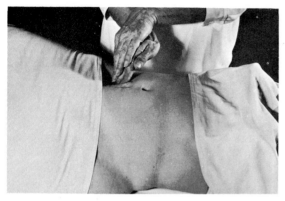

Figure 248

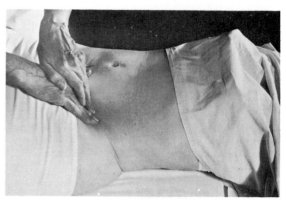

Figure 249

(3) Kneading over the Area of the Colon.

The finger tips of the reinforced right hand are placed about two inches above the area of the distal part of the descending colon (Fig. 250). The finger tips are kept in contact with the skin as in friction movements. A circular movement with firm pressure is repeated several times in this one area and then followed by a firm stroke (Fig. 251) over the area of the distal portion of the colon toward the rectum. With a light stroke, the hand returns to a point about two inches proximal to the starting point and repeats the movements. Progression is made in this manner over the rest of the areas of the descending colon, the transverse colon, and the ascending colon (Fig. 252).

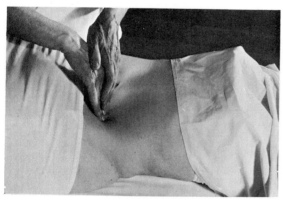

Figure 250

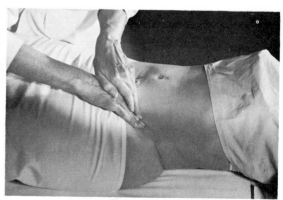

Figure 251

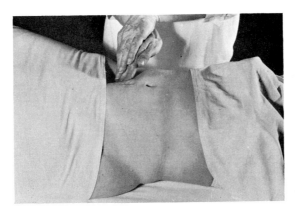

Figure 252

FACE

The therapist stands at the head of the table. The patient is supine.

The following technique for massage of the face is based on the principles of the Hoffa method of massage in that the movements are applied to certain muscles or muscle groups and the stroking movements follow the general longitudinal direction of the muscle fibers.

It must be kept in mind that the muscles of facial expression have little bulk but are thin and located immediately over bony surfaces; therefore the pressure of the massage movements must be very light. This is particularly true when the massage is being given to flaccid muscles that have lost their tone.

This type of massage is particularly applicable in facial paralysis and will aid in preventing and removing fibrosis.

Usually the physician has provided some type of support to the paralyzed muscles between treatments, so as to prevent drooling or to protect the eye.

In general, the movements are from insertion to origin, as indicated by the normal muscle action.

Face (Continued).

Whenever possible, the paralyzed muscles are supported in the position of normal function as the massage is being performed. Support may be given by one hand or fingers of the hand (Figs. 253–260).

Both stroking and kneading are performed with the distal phalanx of the digit(s) used. One or more fingers, either or both thumbs, or thumb and one or more fingers may be used so as to conform to the shape, size, and location of the muscles (Figs. 253–260).

The muscles and muscle groups that are massaged are: frontalis (Fig. 253), orbicularis oculi (Figs. 254, 255), nasalis (Fig. 256), muscles that elevate the corners of the mouth and wrinkle the nose (quadratus labii superior, caninus, zygomaticus, and masseter—Fig. 257), orbicularis oris (Fig. 258), muscles that depress the corners of the mouth (risorius, triangularis, mentalis, and quadratus labii inferiorus—Fig. 259), and platysma (Fig. 260).

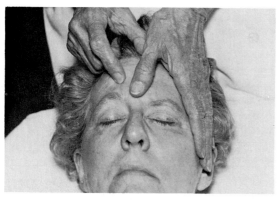

Figure 253

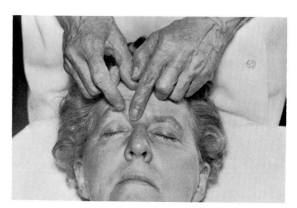

Figure 254

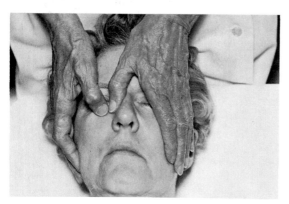

Figure 255

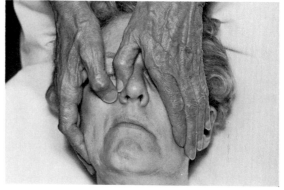

Figure 256

Face (Continued).

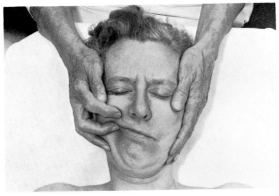

Figure 257

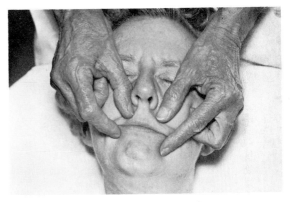

Figure 258

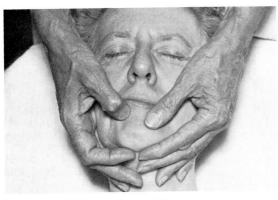

Figure 259

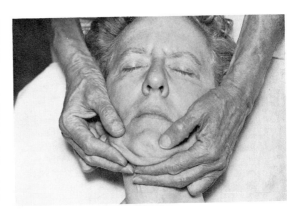

Figure 260

At the finish of the local massage movements to the face, both hands do superficial stroking from the chin to the temples (Fig. 261).

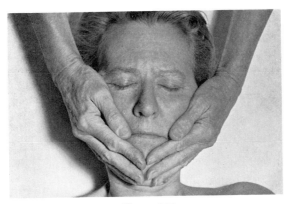

Figure 261

NECK

Note: According to Max Bohm (*Massage, Its Principles and Technic*), Hoffa recommended massage to the sternocleidomastoid muscles for "congestion of the head," its purpose being to stroke over the chief blood vessels and lymphatics of the neck. He considered the origin of the muscle to be at the mastoid process and the insertions at the sternum and clavicle. He stroked and kneaded the muscle from "origin" to "insertion."

MASSAGE IN CHEST PHYSICAL THERAPY

The practice of chest physical therapy in the United States is frequently viewed with much skepticism, criticism and misunderstanding. In Europe the techniques are widely accepted and have been used extensively for many years. Because the American society tends to be so highly "machine" conscious and technically oriented, the physician is inclined to prescribe a "breathing machine" to aid the patient in respiratory distress rather than treat him with physical therapy techniques. Also, if a prescription is sent to a physical therapy department, there may be no physical therapist available who is proficient in respiratory care techniques.

Statistics have shown a consistent increase in the number of chronic obstructive pulmonary disease (C.O.P.D.) patients. During a ten year period (1950–1960) the death rate from emphysema and chronic bronchitis increased more than four times.[12] In an additional study (1950–1965) the mortality rate was shown to double every five years. Deaths increased almost eight times, from 3157 patients in 1950 to 23,700 patients in 1965.[76]

The magnitude of the situation was defined in the following quote. "Chronic obstructive lung disease is rapidly becoming one of the most important health problems of our time".[55] This behooves the health professions to upgrade their understanding and capacity to provide proper treatment. Chest physical therapy (C.P.T.) is attempting to meet these needs in coordination with the other allied health fields.

Chest physical therapy uses physical principles and manual techniques to accomplish the following goals:

1. Prevent the accumulation of secretions.
2. Improve mobilization and drainage of secretions.
3. Instruct patients in home bronchial hygiene programs.
4. Promote relaxation to avoid muscle splinting.
5. Maintain and improve chest wall mobility.
6. Regain the most efficient breathing pattern.
7. Instruct and retrain in use of respiratory muscles.
8. Develop respiratory muscle endurance.
9. Prevent venous stasis.
10. Improve cardiopulmonary exercise tolerance.

When a therapist fully understands these goals, the skepticism and misunderstanding regarding chest physical therapy will be answered.

Chest physical therapy utilizes several techniques to accomplish the above goals: postural drainage, percussion, vibration, facilitation techniques, breathing exercise and retraining, relaxation techniques, posture correction, graded exercise and endurance programs. An in-depth discussion of all of these areas is beyond the limitations of this book. The purpose here is to define and describe the massage techniques used. Therefore percussion and vibration will be presented in detail, and other techniques will be mentioned briefly. Clinical experience* has demonstrated that the coordination of these procedures, in combination with the treatments given by other members (physicians, nurses, and respiration therapists) of the respiratory care service, promotes a unified approach to patient care which is more effective than the application of these techniques as separate treatments.

---

*In the respiratory care service, Wesly Pavilion, Northwestern Memorial Hospital, Chicago, Ill.

Percussion

The technique of clapping or cupping is used as an aid to mobilize secretions which are retained and adherent to the tracheobronchial tree. This percussion sends waves of vibration through the rib cage to the lungs to shake loose adherent mucus plugs in the bronchial tree. (A mucus plug in a segmental bronchus can potentially collapse a lung segment.) Percussion and vibration maneuvers, with the patient in the proper postural drainage position, can help dislodge the plug and facilitate re-expansion of the lung segment or lobe.

Percussion is performed with cupped hands, fingers and thumbs together, the wrists and arms very relaxed and loose. The hands rhythmically and alternately strike the chest wall with emphasis on the area of the lung being drained (see Figs. 262, 263). Cupping of the hands provides a cushion of air between the hands and the chest wall to mechanically deliver a shaking or vibratory movement to the lungs. This technique also serves to prevent unnecessary skin irritation or pain. Skin erythema may be due to several factors. The therapist's hands may not be well-cupped, there may be too much force, or the patient may have an extremely sensitive skin. If the patient prefers, a thin towel, gown or sheet may be placed over the area of treatment. Some patients prefer the treatment directly on the skin to avoid the "shirring" effect which can occur with the use of the covering cloth.

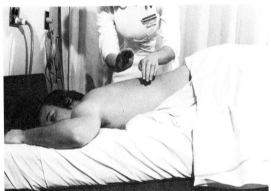

Figure 262

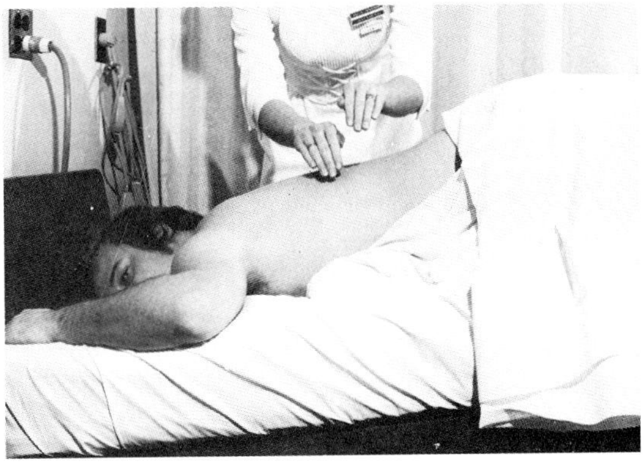

Figure 263

Percussion is quite comfortable when the technique is applied properly; in fact, it has a relaxing effect due to the rhythmicity and consistency of force and direction of movement.

Generally, little force is needed to percuss; it is not force but the cupping that is effective. The force of the percussion must be determined for each patient. For example, different amounts of force would be needed for a child, a large adult, or a patient who had recently had surgery. Conditions such as cystic fibrosis, atelectasis or thick tenacious secretions may need more aggressive chest physical therapy and more percussive force to aid in mobilization of secretions.

The therapist should have a plan for hand movement during percussion so the hands do not wander aimlessly on the patient's thorax. One can work in a circular pattern or up and back laterally, but the pattern should be kept consistent during the treatment. One should not stay in a particular spot for any length of time as this becomes quite irritating. Once skin contact is made, the percussion should continue consistently for approximately three to five minutes, although the time may be varied according to the needs of the individual patient.

Percussion should be applied only over the bony thorax. Care should be taken when percussing anteriorly and at the lateral basilar rib areas since the rib ends are loosely attached or not attached at all (floating ribs). The heel of the hand should not make contact with bony prominences such as the spine of the scapula, clavicles, vertebral column or over developing breast tissue.

GENERAL CONTRAINDICATIONS AND PRECAUTIONS FOR PERCUSSION

1. Flail chest, fractured ribs.
2. Conditions prone to hemorrhage.
3. Conditions in which ribs are fragile, such as metastatic bone cancer and "brittle" bones.
4. Aged and nervous patients who get apprehensive about the procedure.
5. Recent postoperative cases in which pain and muscular splinting would be increased.
6. Subcutaneous emphysema of thorax and neck. The treatment is ineffective since the percussion is absorbed in the subcutaneous layer of air.
7. Unstable cardiac condition.
8. Lung emboli—*Caution*!
9. Recent spinal fusion.
10. Fresh burns, open wounds or infection.

It must be emphasized that the contraindications to postural drainage and percussion and vibration are relative. Priorities must always be considered. For example, if a patient has a poor cardiovascular system that is made worse due to an atelectasis, the atelectasis must be cleared. This situation obviously calls for proper medical judgment, advice and support from the physician.

The indications for percussion are basically the same as for postural drainage. Percussion is routinely done in conjunction with postural drainage (P.D.), especially in patients with thick secretions that are difficult to mobilize. Clinically, it is also seen that respiratory therapy equipment such as the ultrasonic nebulizer or heated aerosol will be of tremendous benefit, especially if given just prior to postural drainage. This form of mist therapy aids in liquefying secretions, making them easier to mobilize.[71] Intermittent positive pressure breathing (IPPB) treatments can also be administered in conjunction with postural drainage, percussion and vibration to distribute air peripherally.[26] This increases the chances of getting air distal to the secretions, making the cough more effective.

Vibration

Vibration is also routinely used with postural drainage (P.D.). It is generally done after or alternating with percussion. The percussion technique is done to loosen the adherent plugs and the vibration to aid in their movement toward the bronchi and trachea, where the secretions can be coughed out or suctioned.

Vibration is performed during the patient's expiratory phase of breathing. The chest is compressed simultaneously with the vibratory movement. Chest compression is extremely important in making vibration effective. The amount of chest compression is determined by several factors, such as chest wall mobility, age of the patient, chest deformities, new postoperative site, chest trauma, fractured ribs. In some cases the therapist may actually perform a "rib springing" technique with the vibration, using a good deal of force in mobilization of the chest wall. Obviously, this is possible only with a mobile thorax.

To accomplish the vibration, the patient is asked to "take a deep breath and blow it all out." Chest compression and vibration are initiated at the peak of inhalation to obtain maximum benefits.

To perform the vibration, the therapist tenses all arm and shoulder muscles in a co-contraction that virtually shakes his own arm and transfers this shaking to the patient's chest wall. (See Figs. 264–271). The vibration is done throughout exhalation. If a more aggressive form of chest compression and vibration (or shaking) is done, the patient takes a deep breath in and the therapist "springs" the ribs in compression three or four times during exhalation.

If the patient is unable to take a deep breath on his own, the intermittent positive pressure breathing (IPPB) treatment or self-inflating bag ("ambu") technique may be used to assist in deep breathing to facilitate the vibration. The vibration technique is performed in the same manner if the IPPB or ambu is used. The patient is mechanically given a large breath and vibration is performed from the peak of inhalation

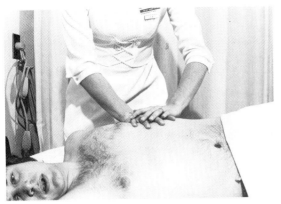

Figure 264

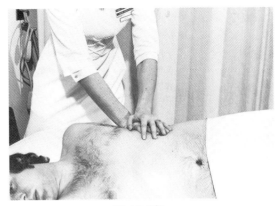

Figure 265

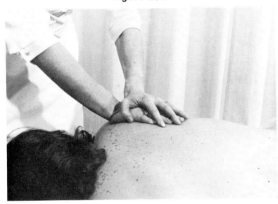

Figure 266

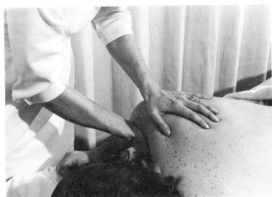

Figure 267

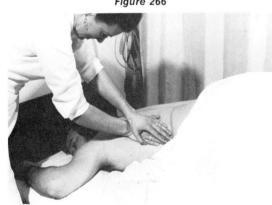

Figure 268

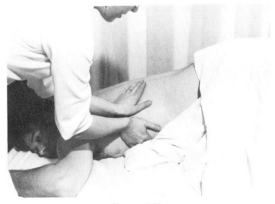

Figure 269

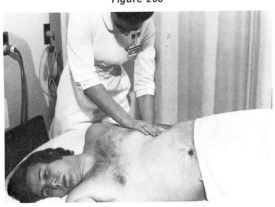

Figure 270

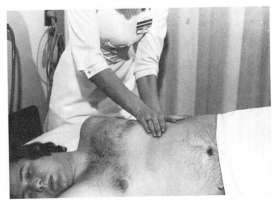

Figure 271

throughout the exhalatory phase. Experience has demonstrated that atelectasis and pneumonias can be cleared more quickly when the ultrasonic nebulizer or heated aerosol is used one half hour prior to the chest physical therapy treatment, whether or not the IPPB or self-inflating bag techniques are used.

The normal cough requires that the patient take a very deep breath, holding it for a few seconds, closing the glottis and vocal cords and building up intrathoracic pressure, then opening glottis and cords and explosively blowing out the air. Patients with a tracheostomy or endotracheal tube cannot cough. The patient with an endotracheal tube cannot cough because the tube passes through the glottis and between the cords, preventing them from closing; the tracheostomized patient has the tube below the cords and thus is unable to build up intrathoracic pressure by closing the glottis and cords. In either case, the major mechanism for clearing secretions has been ablated. One can simulate a "cough" by using the self-inflating bag (with tracheostomy or endotracheal cuff inflated to seal off the airway), giving a large inspiratory volume, holding the bag for two or three seconds, then "popping" the bag open quickly. The therapist begins chest compression and vibration druing the "hold" period of ambu bag inflation and continues throughout the exhalation phase.

There are instances when vibration may be indicated and used even when percussion would not be applicable. Such instances include recent postoperative conditions, open heart surgery, thoracotomies in which pain and splinting would be increased, hemorrhage and fractured ribs. Generally, the same indications, contraindications and precautions are followed as with percussion (see pp. 147–148).

Chest physical therapy has demonstrated its effectiveness in treating the wide spectrum of patients seen in the general hospital physical therapy department. Among these patients are cases of spinal cord injuries, cerebrovascular accidents, myocardial infarctions and neuromuscular disorders. These patients have common respiratory problems: poor ventilation and an ineffective cough. The outcome is retained secretions in the lungs. Many factors contribute to these problems—muscular weakness or paralysis, incoordination, lack of endurance and abnormal habit patterns of breathing.

Debilitated and dependent patients exhibit a marked decrease in activity, even in basic position changes. In a bedridden patient, turning from side to side will effect a general postural drainage of each lung. Gravity becomes both a positive and a negative factor in lung drainage—positive in that the uppermost part of the lung is drained, negative as secretions accumulate in the dependent lobes. Thus, a patient paralyzed on the right side will be more likely to turn to the right side because he has use of the left extremities. He will find it difficult to turn to the left side, and will generally develop a right lung pneumonia. The quadriplegic patient lying on his back will develop a bilateral posterior basal pneumonia or pneumonia in the superior segments of the lower lobes.

The importance of frequent position changes for postural drainage cannot be overemphasized. These frequent changes require a total team effort with the nursing staff.

Neuromuscular disorders such as myasthenia gravis or Guillain-Barré syndrome require assistance also in maintaining or achieving clear lungs so that the patient can fully progress in his rehabilitation. Shortness of breath is caused by secretions in the airways. This is frightening to patients and greatly limits their activity and progress. A program of bronchial hygiene, consisting of postural drainage, percussion, vibration and breathing retraining, should be given prior to exercise. This will allow the patient to tolerate more activity because his airway is clear. There should be a period of rest following bronchial hygiene procedures as they tend to tire the patient.

Patients receiving chest physical therapy pre- and postoperatively have demonstrated fewer respiratory complications and improved postoperative courses of recovery.[27]

To gain expertise in chest physical therapy, therapists not only must be skilled in given percussion and vibration but should also become familiar with postural drainage positions (see pp. 153–159), breathing exercises, exercise programs geared to the patient with respiratory problems, and with other modalities of respiratory therapy. The necessity to integrate and coordinate programs properly becomes obvious as one becomes involved with respiratory care.

appendix 1

CONNECTIVE TISSUE MASSAGE: BINDEGEWEBSMASSAGE

Elizabethe Dicke, a German physical therapist, devised the technique of connective tissue massage in 1929. During a severe and painful illness, primarily with endarteritis obliterans in her right lower extremity for which amputation had been seriously considered, she tried to give herself some relief from backache by stroking over painful areas with the finger tips. She found that such areas were hypersensitive at first, but as the stroking was continued the muscle tension relaxed somewhat, pain eased, and a sensation of warmth in the skin followed. Similar treatment on successive days seemed not only to ease the pain and tension in the back but also to produce some effect on the lower extremity. Sensation began to return, and the skin felt warm, rather than cold. As Frau Dicke continued her self-massage she included stroking around the greater trochanter and along the ilio tibial band. After three months of this massage (done by a colleague), the severe symptoms began to subside. In a year Frau Dicke was back to work as a physical therapist.

Much clinical study and evaluation followed this initial experience. From Frau Dicke's and others' further refinements of her original stroking, and the extension of its use to treating many pathologically involved tissues and organs of the body, the method of "Bindegewebsmassage," now widely used in Europe and especially in Germany by both physicians and physical therapists, has evolved. Broadly speaking, the effects claimed by Frau Dicke and others are that this massage affects the autonomic nervous system and, by reflex action, corrects imbalances in the vegetative functions of the body.

Connective tissue massage has not been generally accepted by physicians and physical therapists in the United States. Very few American doctors and therapists are familiar with this specific method of massage and even fewer are skillful in using it.

Two descriptions of the details of technique and the rationale of the procedures have been written in English and these may be consulted for further information:

Bischof, Irmgard, and Elmiger, Ginette: "Connective Tissue Massage" (Chap. IV in *Massage, Manipulation and Traction* edited by Sidney Licht) Volume V of Physical Medicine Library. Elizabeth Licht, Publisher. New Haven, Conn., 1960.

Ebner, Maria: *Connective Tissue Massage, Theory and Therapeutic Application.* Williams and Wilkins Co., Baltimore, Md., and E. & S. Livingston, Ltd., Edinburgh and London, 1962.

CLOSED-CHEST CARDIAC MASSAGE

This brief description of closed-chest cardiac massage is included as a technique that all physical therapists should know, for prompt use in emergency treatment of cardiac arrest.

If a heart stops beating, as verified by a quick check of the pulse at the carotid arteries on either side of the trachea, the patient should be placed, supine, upon a solid support, such as the floor or a firm plinth or stretcher—whichever is quicker.

The patient's head should be tilted back to assure a patent airway to the lungs.

The heel of one hand, reinforced by the other, is placed just below midsternum. The fingers are spread and raised so that pressure is applied *only to the sternum and not to the ribs or abdomen.* Vertical pressure sufficient to depress the breastbone an inch or a little more is applied and quickly released. This is repeated from 60 to 70 times per minute. If the patient is a child, use one hand and lighter pressure; if a baby, fingers may be used, and much less pressure, with the rate at 80 times per minute.

If there is any assistance available, a physician should be called immediately. The assistant can then administer mouth-to-mouth breathing while closed-chest massage is being done. These measures are continued until the physician arrives or until rigor mortis sets in.

Unless strict care is taken to perform this procedure properly, fractures of the ribs and sternum, and laceration and rupture of soft tissues such as liver, spleen, pancreas, lungs, and blood vessels can easily occur.[43]

appendix 2

POSTURAL DRAINAGE

The use of postural drainage is essential during the percussive and vibration phases of massage for patients with respiratory problems. The therapist must be quite familiar with the proper positioning of patients for draining the various segments and lobes of the lungs.

The line drawings show the use of the tilted bed and pillows for each position, and the positions in which babies may be held on the lap of the mother or therapist. The photographs show the use of pillows alone when the bed cannot be tilted or adjusted.

POSTURAL DRAINAGE—ADULTS

1. APICAL SEGMENTS

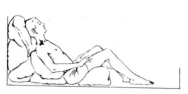

<u>LEFT AND RIGHT ANTERIOR</u>
Sitting — lean back against pillow; clap in front on both sides just above collar bones, between neck and shoulder.

2. APICAL SEGMENTS

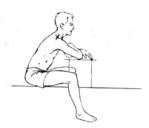

<u>LEFT AND RIGHT POSTERIOR</u>
Sitting — lean forward onto pillow; clap on both sides on the back above shoulder blades. Fingers usually go a little over shoulder.

3. LEFT POSTERIOR SEGMENT

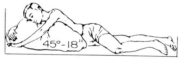

Lie on right side with head and shoulders elevated on pillows. Make 1/4 turn forward; clap over left shoulder blade.

4. APICAL SEGMENTS

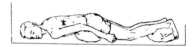

<u>LEFT AND RIGHT (LOWER LOBE)</u>
Lie flat on stomach; place pillow under stomach area for added comfort and clap just below the shoulder blade.

5. RIGHT POSTERIOR SEGMENT

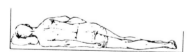

Lie on left side — place pillow in front from shoulder to hips and roll slightly forward onto it; clap over right shoulder blade.

6. ANTERIOR SEGMENTS

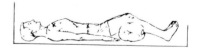

<u>LEFT AND RIGHT</u>
Lie flat on back with pillow under knees for comfort; clap on both sides just below collar bones and above the nipple line.

POSTURAL DRAINAGE — ADULTS

7. RIGHT MIDDLE LOBE

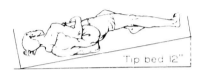

Lie on left side. Place pillow behind from shoulders to hips and roll slightly back onto it; clap over right nipple. For girls developing breast tissue, clap to the right of the nipple and below the armpit.

8. RIGHT LATERAL BASAL SEGMENT

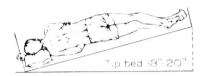

Lie on left side; clap at lower ribs. A pillow under the waist may help to keep the spine straight.

9. POSTERIOR BASAL SEGMENT

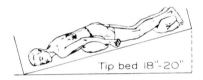

<u>LEFT AND RIGHT</u>
Lie on stomach and place pillow under hips; clap at lower ribs on both sides.

10. LEFT LATERAL BASAL SEGMENT

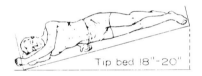

Lie on right side; clap at lower ribs. A pillow under the waist may help to keep spine straight.

11. LEFT LINGULA

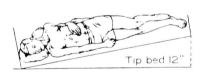

Lie on right side. Place pillow behind from shoulder to hips and roll slightly back onto it; clap over left nipple. For girls developing breast tissue, clap to the left of the nipple and below the armpit.

12. ANTERIOR BASAL SEGMENT

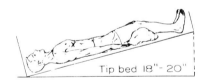

<u>LEFT AND RIGHT</u>
Lie on back and place pillow under knees; clap at lower ribs on both sides.

POSTURAL DRAINAGE—INFANTS

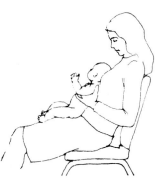

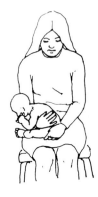

1. APICAL SEGMENTS
LEFT AND RIGHT ANTERIOR
Sitting — lean child back against parent's chest; clap on both sides just above collar bone, between neck and shoulder.

2. APICAL SEGMENTS
LEFT AND RIGHT POSTERIOR
Sitting — lean child forward onto pillow or arm; clap on both sides on the back above the shoulder blades. Fingers go a little over the shoulders.

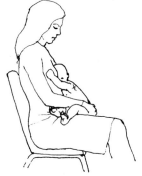

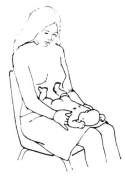

3. LEFT POSTERIOR SEGMENT
Place child on lap facing to the right. Lean him against parent so that the chest of the child is against the upper portion of the parent's body. Clap over left shoulder blade.

4. APICAL SEGMENTS (LOWER LOBE)
LEFT AND RIGHT SIDES
Place child on stomach. Clap just below the shoulder blades.

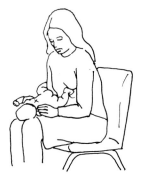

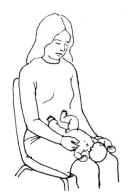

5. RIGHT POSTERIOR SEGMENT
Place child on left side. Support him with the right hand around his upper right arm. Roll him slightly forward onto parent's right arm. Clap over right shoulder blade.

6. ANTERIOR SEGMENTS
LEFT AND RIGHT
Place child on back. Clap just below the collar bone and above the nipple line.

POSTURAL DRAINAGE—INFANTS

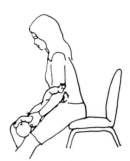

7. RIGHT MIDDLE LOBE
Extend left leg. Place child on his left side in head down position. Support his upper right arm with parent's left hand. Roll him slightly back onto parent's left arm. Clap over right nipple.

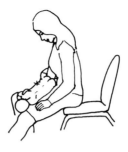

8. RIGHT LATERAL BASAL SEGMENT
Extend left leg. Place child on his left side in head down position. Support his right upper arm with parent's right hand. Clap at lower ribs.

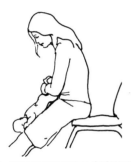

9. POSTERIOR BASAL SEGMENT LEFT TO RIGHT
Extend both legs. Place child on stomach in head down position. Clap at lower ribs on both sides.

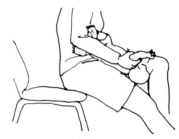

10. LEFT LINGULA
Extend right leg. Place child on his right side in head down position. Support his upper right arm with parent's right hand. Roll him slightly back onto parent's right arm. Clap over left nipple.

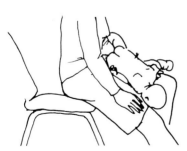

11. LEFT LATERAL BASAL SEGMENT
Extend right leg. Place child on his right side in head down position. Support his left upper arm with parent's left hand. Clap at lower ribs.

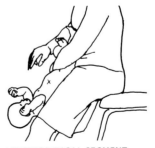

12. ANTERIOR BASAL SEGMENT LEFT AND RIGHT
Extend both legs. Place child on back in head down position. Clap at lower ribs on both sides.

*Use of pillows to achieve proper position of patient,
on bed or table in the hospital, the clinic, or at home*

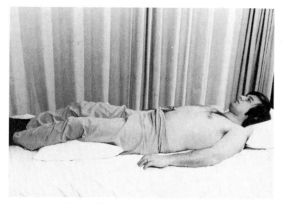

1. Upper lobes—anterior segments

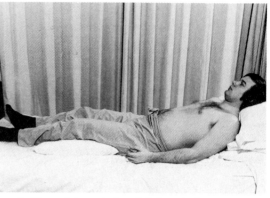

2. Upper lobes—left and right apical segments

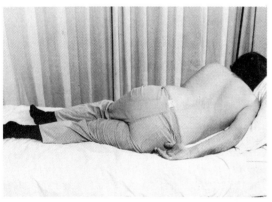

3. Left upper lobe—posterior segment

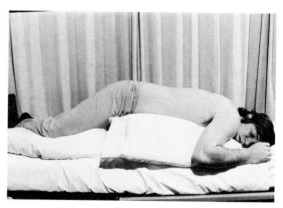

4. Right upper lobe—posterior segment

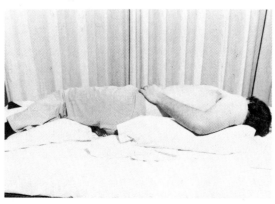

5. Left upper lobe—lingular segment

*Use of pillows to achieve proper position of patient,
on bed or table in the hospital, the clinic, or at home.*

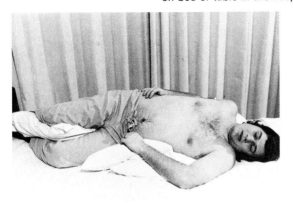

6. *Right middle lobe*

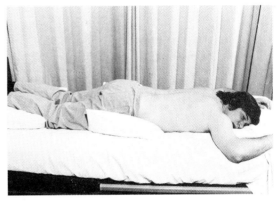

7. *Left and right lower lobes—apical segments*

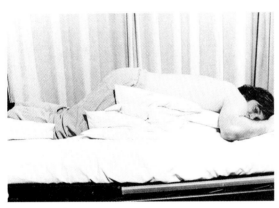

8. *Left and right lower lobes—posterior segments**

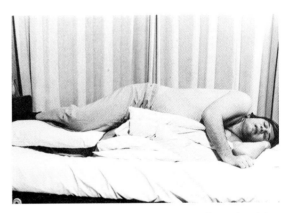

9. *Right lower lobe—lateral segment. Opposite sidelying for left lower lobe—lateral segment.*

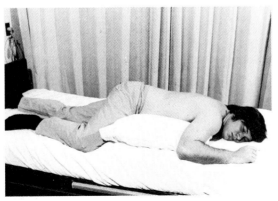

10. *Modified ¾ prone position to drain posterior
basilar segments.*

---

*Left and right lower lobes—anterior segments: patient would lie supine instead of prone; same pillow arrangement, with hips elevated and head and shoulders lower.

bibliography

1. American College of Surgeons: An Outline of the Treatment of Fractures. Chicago, Committee on Fractures, 1940.
2. Barr, J. S., and Taslitz, N.: Influence of back massage on autonomic functions. Physical Therapy, J. of A.P.T.A. 50:1679–1691, 1970.
3. Beard, G.: History of massage technique. Phys. Ther. Rev., 32:613–624, 1952.
4. Bell, A. J.: Massage and the physiotherapist. Physiotherapy 50:406–408, 1964.
5. Bendixen, H. H., Egbert, L. D., Hedley-White, J., Laver, M. B., and Pontoppidan, H.: Respiratory Care. St. Louis, C. V. Mosby, 1965, pp. 99–101.
6. Berghman, G., and Helleday, U.: Anteckningar om massage. Nordiskt Medicinskt Arkin. 5:No. 7, 1873.
7. Bodian, M.: Use of massage following lid surgery. Eye, Ear, Nose and Throat Monthly 48:542–47, 1969.
8. Bohm, M.: Massage—Its Principles and Technic. Philadelphia, Chas. F. Saunders, 1918.
9. Bork, K., Karling, G. W., Faust, G.: Serum enzyme levels after "whole body massage." Arch. Dermatol. Forsch. 240:324–48, 1971.
10. Brunton, T. L., and Tunnicliffe, T. W.: On the effects of the kneading of muscles upon the circulation, local and general. J. Physiol. 17:364, 1894–1895.
11. Bucholz, C. H.: Therapeutic Exercise and Massage. Philadelphia, Lea & Febiger, 1917, p.130.
12. Carey, F. E.: Emphysema. The Battle to Breathe. U. S. Dept. of H.E.W., Public Service Health Publication #1715, 1967, p. 1–3.
13. Carrier, E. B.: Studies on physiology of capillaries; reaction of human skin capillaries to drugs and other stimuli. Am. J. Physiol. 61:528–547, 1922.
14. Cherniak, R. M., Cherniak, L., and Naimark, A.: Respiration in Health and Disease. (2nd ed.) Philadelphia, W. B. Saunders, 1972, p.452.
15. Chor, H., and Dolkart, R. E.: A study of simple disuse atrophy in the monkey. Am. J. Physiol. 117:4, 1936.
16. Chor, H., Cleveland, D., Davenport, H. A., Dolkart, R. E., and Beard, G.: Atrophy and regeneration of the gastrocnemius-soleus muscles: Effects of physical therapy in monkey following section and suture of sciatic nerve. J.A.M.A. 113:1029–1033, 1939.
17. Clark, D. T.: Complications following closed-chest cardiac massage. J.A.M.A. 181:337-338, 1962.
18. Cleoburey, W.: System of Friction. (3rd ed.) London, Munday & Slatter, 1825.
19. Coulter, J. S.: Clio Medica VII, Physical Therapy. New York, Paul B. Hoeber, 1932, pp. 39–40.
20. Cuthbertson, D. P.: Effect of Massage on Metabolism: A survey. Glasgow M. J. (New 7th Series) 2:200–213, 1933.
21. Cyriax, J.: Treatment by Massage and Manipulation. New York, Paul Hoeber, Inc., 1959.
22. Despard, L. L.: Textbook of Massage and Remedial Gymnastics, (3rd ed.) New York, Oxford University Press, 1932.
23. Downing, George: The Massage Book. New York, Random House. The Bookworks, 1972.
24. Drinker, C. K., and Yoffey, J. M.: Lymphatics, Lymph. and Lymphoid Tissue: Their Physiological and Clinical Significance. Cambridge, Harvard University Press. 1941, p. 310.
25. Ebner, M.: Connective Tissue Massage, Theory and Therapeutic Application. Edinburgh and London, E. & S. Livingston Ltd., 1962.
26. Egan, D. F.: Fundamentals of Inhalation Therapy. St. Louis, C. V. Mosby 1969, p.206, 406.
27. Egbert, L. D., Battit, G. E., Welch, C. E., and Bartlett, M. K.: Reduction of postoperative pain by encouragement and instruction of patients. New Eng. J. Med. 270:825–827, 1964.
28. Galen, C.: De Sanitate Tuenda (a translation of Galen's Hygiene by R. M. Green). Springfield, Ill., Charles C Thomas, 1951.
29. Graham, D.: Practical Treatise on Massage. New York, Wm. Wood and Co., 1884.
30. Graham, D.: Massage—Manual Treatment and Remedial Movements. Philadelphia, J. B. Lippincott, 1913.
31. Granit, R.: Receptors and Sensory Perception. New Haven, Yale University Press, 1955, pp. 191–276.
32. Hartman, F. A., Blatz, W. E., and Kelborn, L. J.: Studies in regeneration of denervated mammalian muscle. Am. J. Physiol. 53:109, 1919.
33. Hartman, F. A., and Blatz, W. E.: Treatment of Denervated muscle. J.A.M.A. 74:878, 1920.
34. Hoffa, A.: Tecknik der Massage. Stuttgart, Verlag Von Ferdinand Ernke, 1897.
35. Johnson, W.: The Anatriptic Art. London, Simkin Marshall and Co., 1866.
36. Kalb, S. W.: The fallacy of massage in the treatment of obesity. J. Med. Soc. N. J. 41:406–407, 1944.
37. Kellgren, A.: The Technic of Ling's System of Manual Treatment. Edinburgh and London, Young J. Pentland, 1890.
38. Kellogg, J. H.: The Art of Massage. (12th ed., revised.) Battle Creek, Mich., Modern Medical Publishing Co., 1919.
39. Key, J. A., Elzinga, E., and Fischer, F.: Local atrophy of bone, I. Effect of immobilization and of operative procedures. Arch. Surg. 28:935–942, 1934.
40. Key, J. A., Elzinga, E., and Fischer, F.: Local atro-

phy of bone, II. Effects of local heat, massage, and therapeutic exercise. Arch. Surg. *28*:943–947,1934.

41. Kleen, E. A. G.: Handbook I Massage och Sjukgymnastik. Stockholm, Nordin and Josephson, 1906.

42. Kleen, E. A. G.: Massage and Medical Gymnastics. (2nd ed.) New York, Wm. Wood and Co., 1921.

43. Kouwenhoven, W. D., Jude, J. R., and Knickerbocker, G. G.: Closed-chest cardiac massage. J.A.M.A., *173*:1064–1067, 1960.

44. Krusen, F. H.: Physical Medicine, Philadelphia, W. B. Saunders Co., 1941, p. 335.

45. Ladd, M. P., Kottke, F. J., and Blanchard, R. S.: Studies of the effect of massage on the flow of lymph from the foreleg of the dog. Arch. Phys. Med. *33*:611, 1952.

46. Langley, J. N., and Hashimoto, M.: Denervated muscle atrophy. Am. J. Physiol. *52*:15, 1918.

47. LeRoy, M. R.: La vie du tissu conjuntife et sa defense par la massage. Rev. Med. Paris *58*:212, 1941.

48. Lewis, T.: Blood Vessels of Human Skin and Their Responses. London, Shaw & Sons, Ltd., 1927, pp. 128, 233.

49. Licht, S. (ed.): Massage, Manipulation and Traction. New Haven, Elizabeth Licht, 1960, pp. 29–31, 41, 57–69, 131–132.

50. Lucia, S. P., and Rickard, J. F.: Effects of massage on blood platelet production. Proc. Soc. Exper. Biol. Med. *31*:87, 1933.

51. Maggiora, A.: De l' action physiologique du massage sur les muscles de l' homme. Arch. Ital. Biol. *16*:225, 1891.

52. McMaster, P. D.: Changes in the cutaneous lymphatics of human beings and in the lymph flow under normal and pathological conditions. J. Exper. Med. *65*:347, 1937.

53. McMillan, M.: Massage and Therapeutic Exercise. Philadelphia, W. B. Saunders Co., 1925.

54. Mennell, J. B.: Physical Treatment. (5th ed.) Philadelphia, Blakiston Co., 1945.

55. Miller, W. F.: Rehabilitation of patients with chronic obstructive lung disease. Med. Clin. N. Amer. *51*:349, 1967.

56. Mitchell, J. K.: Massage and Exercise in System of Physiologic Therapeutics. Philadelphia, Blakiston's Sons & Co., 1904, pp. 20–21, 56.

57. Mock, H. E.: Massage in surgical cases, in A.M.A. Handbook of Physical Medicine, Council of Physical Medicine, A.M.A. Chicago, 1945, p. 95.

58. Murrell, W.: Massage as a Mode of Treatment. London, H. K. Lewis, 1886.

59. Nordschow, M., and Bierman, W.: Influence of manual massage on muscle relaxation: effect on trunk flexion. J. Am. Phys. Ther. Assoc. *42*:653, 1962.

60. Pemberton, R.: Physiology of massage. In A.M.A. Handbook of Physical Therapy. (3rd ed.) Chicago, Council of Physical Therapy A.M.A., 1939, pp. 78–87.

61. Pemberton, R.: Physiology of massage. In A.M.A. Handbook of Physical Medicine. Council of Physical Medicine, A.M.A. Chicago, 1945, p. 141

62. Pemberton, R.: Physiology of massage. In A.M.A. Handbook of Physical Medicine and Rehabilitation. Philadelphia and Toronto, Blakiston Co., 1950, p. 133.

63. Pemberton, R.: The physiologic influence of massage and the clinical application of heat and massage in internal medicine. In Principles and Practices of Physical Medicine, Vol. I. Hagerstown, Md., W. F. Prior Co., 1932.

64. Reiter, S., Garrett, T. R., and Erickson, D. J.: Current trends in the use of therapeutic massage. Jour. A.P.T.A. *49*:158–161, 1969.

65. Ruch, T. C., and Fulton, J. F.: Medical Physiology and Biophysics. (18th ed.) Philadelphia, W. B. Saunders Co., 1960, pp. 167–205, 253–264, 350–367, 694–703, 738–741.

66. Schneider, E. C., and Havens, L. C.: Changes in the blood flow after muscular activity and during Training. Am. J. Physiol. *36*:259, 1915.

67. Severini, V., and Venerando, A.: The physiological effects of massage on the cardiovascular system. Europa Medicophys. *3*:165–183, 1967.

68. Severini, V., and Venerando, A.: Effect on the peripheral circulation of substances producing hyperemia in combination with massage. Europa Medicophys. *3*:184–198, 1967.

69. Suskind, M. I., Hajek, N. A., and Hines, H. M.: Effects of massage on denervated skeletal muscle. Arch. Phys. Med., *27*:133–135, 1946.

70. Tappan, F.: Massage Techniques. A Case Method Approach, New York, Macmillan Co., 1961.

71. Thacker, W. E.: Postural Drainage and Respiratory Control. London, Lloyd-Luke, 1965, p.20.

72. Thomas's Medical Dictionary. Philadelphia, J. B. Lippincott Co., 1886.

73. Wakim, K. G.: The effects of massage on the circulation in normal and paralyzed extremities. Arch. Phys. Med. *30*:135, 1949.

74. Wakim, K. G.: Influence of centripetal rhythmic compression on localized edema of an extremity. Arch. Phys. Med. *36*:98, 1955.

75. Watkins, A.: Physical Medicine in General Practice. Philadelphia, J. B. Lippincott Co., 1946, p. 39.

76. Weiss, E. B., et al.: Acute respiratory failure in chronic obstructive lung disease (Part I, Pathophysiology), In Dowling, H. F.: D. M. Disease-a-Month. Chicago, Year Book Medical Publishers, 1969, (October) p.3.

77. Wide, A.: Handbook of Medical and Orthopedic Gymnastics. (3rd ed.) New York, Funk & Wagnalls Co., 1905.

78. Wolfson, H.: Studies on effect of physical therapeutic procedures on function and structure. J.A.M.A., *96*:2020, 2021, 1931.

79. Wood, E. C., Kosman, A. J., and Osborne, S. L.: Effects of massage upon denervated skeletal muscles of the dog. Phys. Ther. Rev., *28*:284–285, 1948.

80. Wright, J.: The prescription of physical therapy. Phys. Ther. Rev., *26*:168–169, 1946.

81. Wright, S.: Physiological aspects of rheumatism. Proc. Roy. Soc. Med., *32*:651–662, 1939.

82. Wright, V. W. M.: Practical fracture physical therapy. Surg. Clin. N. Amer., *17*:1683–1703, 1937.

83. Yoffey, J. M., and Courtice, F. C.: Lymphatics, Lymph and Lymphoid Tissue. London, Edward Arnold, 1956, p. 324.

84. Zabludowski, J. B: Technique of Massage. Leipzig, G. Thieme, 1903.

index